OUR LADY of WEIGHT LOSS

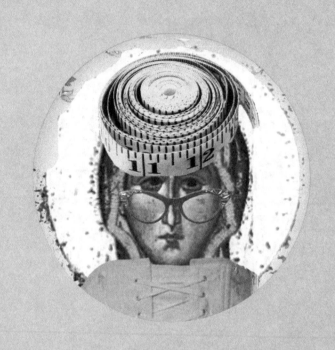

OUR LADY of WEIGHT LOSS

Miraculous and Motivational Musings
from the Patron Saint
of Permanent Fat Removal

JANICE TAYLOR

Viking Studio

VIKING STUDIO

Published by the Penguin Group

Penguin Group (USA) Inc, 375 Hudson Street, New York, New York 10014, U.S.A. · Penguin Group (Canada), 90 Eglinton Avenue East, Suite 700, Toronto, Ontario, Canada M4P 2Y3 (a division of Pearson Penguin Canada Inc.) · Penguin Books Ltd, 80 Strand, London WC2R 0RL, England · Penguin Ireland, 25 St. Stephen's Green, Dublin 2, Ireland (a division of Penguin Books Ltd) · Penguin Books Australia Ltd, 250 Camberwell Road, Camberwell, Victoria 3124, Australia (a division of Pearson Australia Group Pty Ltd) · Penguin Books India Pvt Ltd, 11 Community Centre, Panchsheel Park, New Delhi – 110 017, India · Penguin Group (NZ), Cnr Airborne and Rosedale Roads, Albany, Auckland 1310, New Zealand (a division of Pearson New Zealand Ltd) · Penguin Books (South Africa) (Pty) Ltd, 24 Sturdee Avenue, Rosebank, Johannesburg 2196, South Africa

Penguin Books Ltd, Registered Offices: 80 Strand, London WC2R 0RL, England

First published in 2006 by Viking Studio, a member of Penguin Group (USA) Inc.

Illustrations by the author

Publisher's Note: Neither the publisher nor the author is engaged in rendering professional advice or services to the individual reader. The ideas, procedures, and suggestions contained in this book are not intended as a substitute for consulting with your physician. All matters regarding your health require medical supervision. Neither the author nor the publisher shall be liable or responsible for any loss or damage allegedly arising from any information or suggestion in this book.

ISBN 0-14-200508-8

Printed in the United States of America
Set in Joanna
Designed by Chris Welch

This book is dedicated to my mother, Harriet Taylor,
Our Lady of Gracious Pastry,

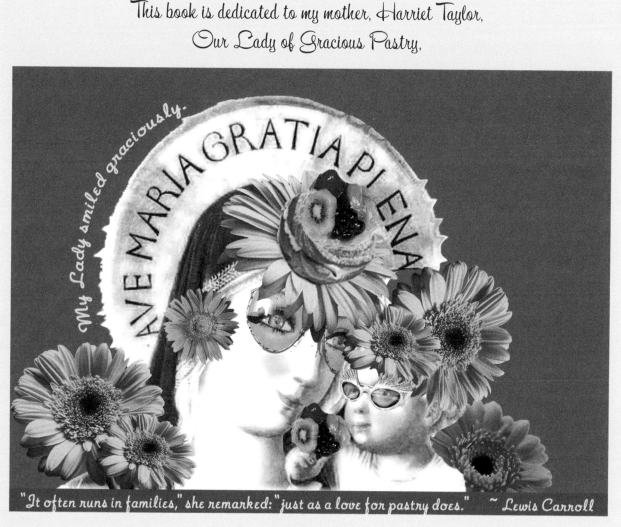

as well as to the kindly nuns from
the Convent of Our Lady of Snow, Blue Point, New York.

Acknowledgments

Deepest and most sincere thanks and gratitude to those who supported me in a multitude of ways.

First and foremost, heaping platters of gratitude to my husband, best friend, and art director, Peter, who has many opinions (usually helpful) and who thankfully does not eat in front of me post-9 P.M. Joshua, my son, for appreciating my artistic nature, for his dry wit, wisdom, and professional counsel. Abby, my daughter, who always has an encouraging word and creative idea and who sweetly and softly spreads the Our Lady of Weight Loss word. My mother, Harriet, who reigns supreme. My father, Benjamin, who is with me in spirit. Love and thanks to my sister, brothers, and Praise Be! my New York and Chicago cousins—Jane, Larry, Alan, Maeve, Jeanette, Angus, Lesley, David, Nancy, Amy, George, Gloria, Sue, Jesse, Dave, Jill— and Uncle Sy, and, of course!, my mother-in-law, Sarah.

Thanks to Megan Graves, whose beauty, both inside and out, inspires. Tommy Hansen and Daria Panichas, whose generosity in time, spirit, and expertise will always be greatly appreciated. Anna J. Allen, who got it immediately and never let go. Carole Goldstein, my secret weapon. Kathy Cano Murillo (The Crafty Chica), whose generosity blows me over. Jane Weston Wilson, my friend, mentor, and role model.

Thanks to Jay Kriegel, for the seventeen-year thrill ride (the apprentice becomes the master). Jim Abernathy, Adam Miller, who supported me more than they may realize, Ernesto Aguilar, Mary Ann De Jesus, Matthew Pritchard, Carl Garris, Michael Walker, and Edwin Nazario.

Thanks to Pam Roule, Abigail Roule, Wendy Levinson, Dana Levinson, Andrew Levinson, Evan Mahl, Angelica Canales, Kate Severin, Lissa Weinmann, John Loggia, Aimee Leone, Kathy Mancuso, Vick Vats, Lisa Bisagni, Steve Bernstein, Anita Gonzales, Holly Ventura, Arlene Parks, David Mahl, Ron Roth, Jeanne McManus, Roland Rameshwar, Leslie Jacobs-McIntosh, Mary Margaret Hansen, Lisa Fedich, June Kosloff, Deborah Drucker, Lindsey Roth-Rosen, Rosemary Zraly (The Champagne Lady), Debra Hastings, Tina Zaremba, Michael Higgins, Gwynne Philbrook, Amy Stanton, Stephanie Jo Klein (Klein Creative Communications), Marita Florini, Cathy Kerila, Frank Furgal, Gina Fuentes-Walker, Reuben Sinha, and the Time Paradox Group.

Thanks to Wade Schields, Craig Stodola, Stephanie Sloane, Judy Temes, Jami Bernard, Susyn Reeve, Bev Bennett, Dee Adams, Marilynn Preston, Jaime Sarrio, Wendy Korn, Patricia Kitchen, Paula Wilkerson, Kelly Love Johnson, Farrah Weinstein, Iyna Bort Caruso, Eva Fellows, Lindsey Lusiak, Christina Coppa, Danny Evans, Claudia H. Christian, Julia Dahl, Melissa Statmore, Kathryn Compton, Margaret Jawkowski, Nancy Galyon, Joseph Giardino, Joe Valentino, Clare Probert, Margaret Magnarelli, Raakhee Mirchandani, Colette Bouchez, Laura Fenamore, Julie Ridl (The Daily Skinny Post), Karen Post (The Branding Diva),

Aryeh Hecht (Vitalicious Muffins), Julia Cameron, Emma Lively, Cindy Adams, and Simon Doonan.

Special thanks to Debra Goldstein, my amazing agent, Elizabeth Little and all at The Creative Culture. My brilliant editor, Lucia Watson, and to those at Viking Studio who made this a joyous experience—Megan Newman, Kate Stark, Lissa Brown, Jessica Lee, Rebecca Behan, Molly Brouillette, Grace Veras, Amy Hill, and Carla Bolte. Thanks to Neil Burstein, Esq., Marcela Landres, editorial consultant, and to Olga Kogan, linguistic specialist.

Thanks to Kandji Medoune, the best cabbie in New York City, who predicted, with great enthusiasm, a very positive future for Our Lady of Weight Loss. What a ride!

And to all Our Lady's Kick in the Tush Club members and fans who generously contributed their letters, their weighty confessions, and encouraged me. And to everyone and anyone who has purchased my art, uttered a kind word, smiled, nodded, made any kind of positive gesture in my direction . . . you'll never know how these acts of kindness affect one.

Contents

OUR LADY of WEIGHT LOSS

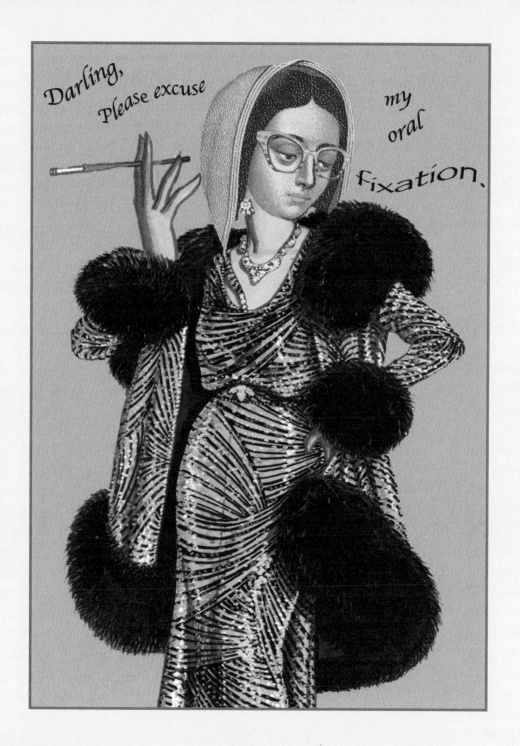

The Ten Commandments
of
Permanent Fat Removal

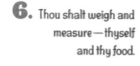

1. Thou shalt honor and believe in thyself.

2. Thou shalt move thy booty. Move it and move it some more.

3. Thou shalt never go hungry again. Eat small meals and healthy snacks throughout the day.

4. Thou shalt stock thy fridge with the right stuff—the fruits and vegetables of the earth.

5. Thou shalt honestly write it down. If you bite it. you must write it.

6. Thou shalt weigh and measure—thyself and thy food.

7. Thou shalt drink enough Holy Water to frighten Noah and map out all the restrooms in thy village.

8. Thou shalt not deny thyself a treat or two now and then.

9. Thou shalt not eat out of misery. boredom. anxiety … but should thou indulge. thou shalt forgive thyself.

10. Thou shalt not covet thy neighbor's plate.

The Arrival of Our Lady of Weight Loss

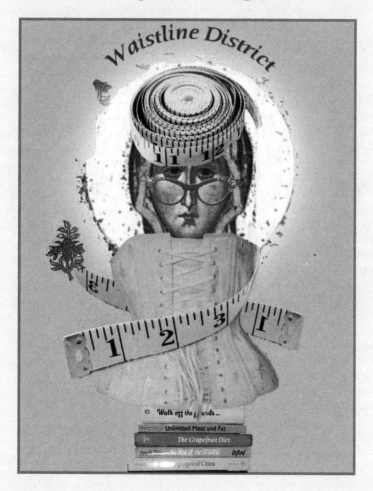

> "The journey of a thousand miles must begin with a single step."
> ~ Chinese proverb

faᴛoid

Nearly two thirds
of adults in the United
States are overweight,
and 30.5 percent
are obese.

Before we begin, I would like to be completely up front about the fact that I'm not here to tell you how to lose weight and keep it off. I own so many diet books myself that I once thoughtfully labeled a certain area of my office the "Watch Your Waistline District." My hope was that there was enough fat-burning power in the combined mass of words alone that a mere visit to this zone would prove sufficient to remove fat. It did not work.

I have yo-yoed (an athletic feat, performed gracefully) ten pounds up, twenty down; five up, thirty-five down; fifty up—in short, enough pounds to equal ten people. I know how it feels to go from being a full-fledged hog, dumping the contents of the refrigerator down the hatch in the space of thirty seconds, to chewing low-cal, low-fat, dainty cucumber sandwiches (hold the mayo) slowly and deliberately, as Zen macrobiotic diets suggest. The Zen theory is that chewing one hundred times per spoonful increases awareness, mindfulness, and digestion. Truthfully, I've never made it past thirty chews before my mind wandered off, but I am nevertheless proud of my thirty-chew accomplishment.

I know the siren cry of almighty food well. (I hear the biscotti right now. It's only 20 calories and 0 fat grams per piece, yet it calls.) I know the humiliation of broken zippers and split pants. And I know the victory of taking pounds off, and the beauty and glow of being svelte.

But it wasn't until Our Lady of Weight Loss entered my life that I was able to permanently remove more than fifty pounds of my own excess baggage.

Our Lady Appears

Our Lady of Weight Loss first made her presence known to me during one of those group meetings where everyone obsesses about food and weight.

I'd dragged myself to the weight-loss center because, while dressing that morning, I made the "mistake" of standing in front of a full-length mirror as I pulled up my XXL elastic-band pants. Oh, my—describing them as tight doesn't even do it justice! At that moment a line was drawn in the sand (well, literally an elastic waistband line had been drawn upon my stomach). Buying XXXL pants was not an option. At some point they, too, would become tight. And if I were to be totally honest with myself, which I uncharacteristically was on that particular morning, there were a multitude of other reasons why I should lose weight. My back hurt a good deal of the time, my cholesterol was over 250, and I had to wear orthotics in my shoes, which meant no slinky sandals or heels.

In essence, I was five minutes to never sexy.

The Voice

So there I was at yet another meeting, about to embark on yet another diet. As I weighed in and joined the thirty or so other women

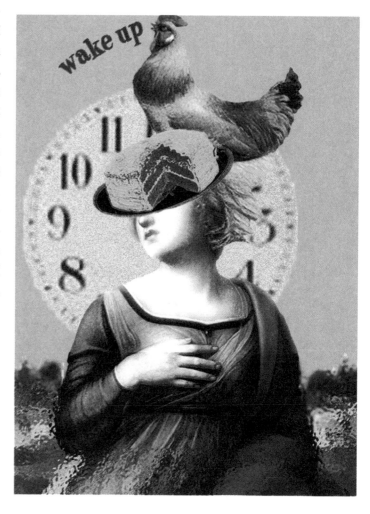

for the lecture, tears came to my eyes. I thought about how far I had to go and how many times I had traveled the same dreary, depressing road of deprivation. I thought, "I'm never going to make it."

That's when I heard The Voice. She said, "If you think you're never going to make it, you never will." Needless to say, I was a bit taken aback, but I had to give credence to The Voice. She had a valid point. I wondered where The Voice was coming from, and quickly concluded that it was too wise to be coming from me, as I was way too mired in self-pity to think of anything constructive on my own. The Voice continued, "You're an artist. Make weight loss an art project." It was as though I had been hit with a Zen stick. I was awakened.

Now alert, my attention shifted back to the meeting, as the group leader was exuberantly extolling the virtues of red peppers. "Juicy, refreshing, colorful," she said. That's when inspiration hit.

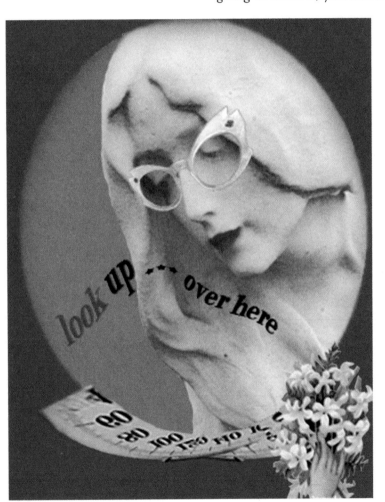

look up ... over here

Tasty Tidbit **What is a Zen stick? A Zen stick is something that a Zen master hits their student with in order to jolt them out of their semi-unconscious state into an awakened one.**

Our Lady of Weight Loss Is in the House!

I went home and headed straight into my studio. I lit a candle (a common practice), called upon The Voice to guide me (an uncommon practice), opened my heart and soul, and released any preconceived notions of how to make art and lose weight at the same time (an interesting combo). At first, it didn't seem to make sense, But with visions of sexy vegetables dancing through my head, I began cutting and pasting as I asked her for help.

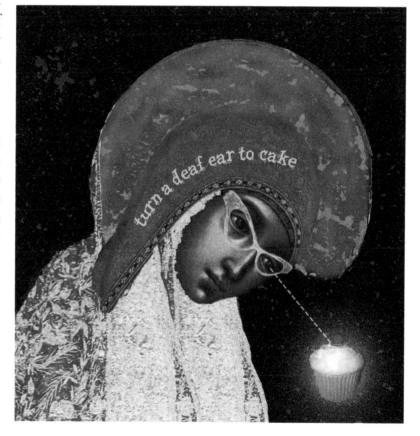

Hi Voice. Thanks for whispering such inspiring and comforting thoughts in my ear this morning. I'm following your suggestions and making weight loss an art project. I'm not exactly sure where I'm headed, so I'm thinking I could use some help. I've been uncomfortable asking for help in the past, so this is new for me, but it feels good to put it right out there. If you feel like working on these collages with me, please feel free to toss your ideas my way. You can either whisper to me again, let images serendipitously come my way, or do the cutting and pasting yourself. I hereby relinquish control to you. Thank you!
~Janice

As I worked on these collages, my mind wandered back to childhood—a memory no doubt triggered by the combination of scissors and Elmer's Glue.

Our Lady of Snow

When I was young, my dad owned a small-town pharmacy and my mom and I would make deliveries for him. My favorite stop was the

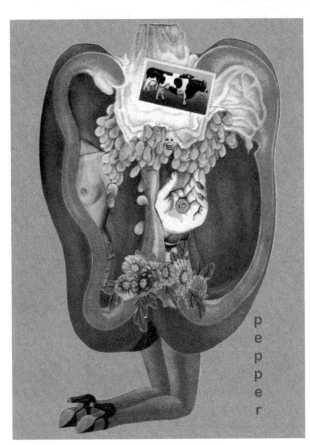

Convent of Our Lady of Snow. The nuns were always kind to me. They would say, "Aren't you a pretty girl—so good to help your mother," as they kindly patted my head. They never made mention of my size, as many others did, nor did they make the comment I'd gotten used to hearing: "What a shame. You have such a pretty face."

As I cut and pasted my way through my first weight-loss collage, I remembered the beautiful statue of Our Lady of Snow that stood at the convent's entrance. Surely, I thought, there must be a patron saint for permanent fat removal.

At the end of the day, the first of the sexy vegetable series—*Ms. Red Pepper*—was standing before me. The same feelings of warmth, acceptance, love, and peace that I had felt when the nuns patted my head washed over me. I smiled and said aloud, "Our Lady of Weight Loss. I know you're here."

I'd always traveled the weight-loss trail on my own. But this time I set off on the rocky road to Svelteville with my art supplies in hand and Our Lady of Weight Loss by my side.

No longer alone, I had the best possible companion and a new faith—in both her and in me. This time would be *the* time.

The Fat Exchange

As the weeks and months passed, I collaged, sewed, and crocheted my way through mountains of cakes, cookies, candies, and fries. Instead of eating these tempting treats, I made art about them. In the process, I exchanged over fifty pounds of excess weight for fifty pieces of art.

With each stitch or swath of paste and paper, I spoke to myself (and Our Lady) as my relationship with food began to change.

Hi Our Lady! *Take a look at this. I just sewed a piece of Chocolate Fudge Chip Cake. When I see cake, I no longer think about eating it. I chew over (ha!) how I might make patterns in the icing when I sew it! I am beginning to equate "dieting" (there must be a better word for it) with pleasure. What's happening here?* ~Janice

I realized that with Our Lady of Weight Loss at my side, I could redirect the feeding frenzy.

I had always given food way too much power. Making art about food wasn't just a distraction, it was a way to embrace food—to stare down the enemy and learn how to befriend it and play with it.

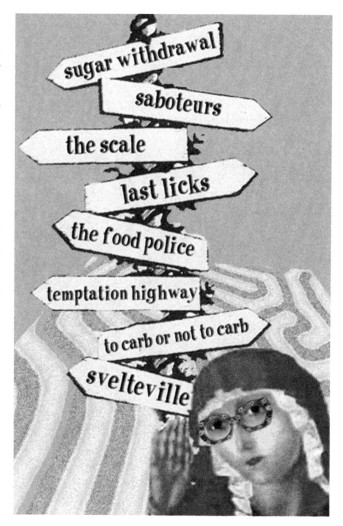

sugar withdrawal
saboteurs
the scale
last licks
the food police
temptation highway
to carb or not to carb
svelteville

Since that very first day, Our Lady's been at my side, and I've undergone a dramatic change. It's not just my body that's different. My hair (big and bouncy, with ridiculously expensive highlights—don't even ask), my glasses (funkiest ever), my clothing (formfitting), and my attitude (don't mess with me!) have all been transformed.

Our Lady Is Here for You, Too!

Our Lady of Weight Loss is here for you, too, and she has instructed me to pass on the basics of what she deems the most important aspects of permanent fat removal.

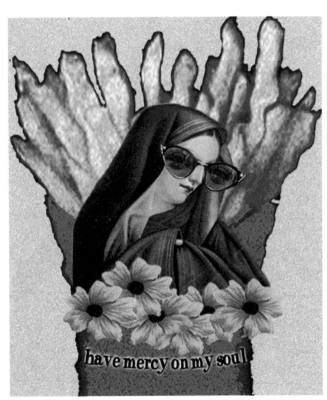

Our Lady's basic philosophy is this: All diets work, if you follow them. However, she's noticed that there are many of us who have a modicum of difficulty (she's being kind) when it comes to sticking to a long-term, healthy life plan.

She understands that a sound food plan is crucial. Sorry, you can't eat unlimited amounts of deep-fried Oreos. Our Lady's theory is that if you take a lighthearted, creative approach to weight loss and focus on your breath, your thoughts, and the simple pleasures and joys of life you will have a much easier and happier time sticking to whatever food plan or healthy lifestyle you've mapped out for yourself.

Our Lady of Weight Loss wants to share her philosophy and her "weigh" with you. So, she dictated this book. That's right—all her wisdom is here. (My transcription skills leave much to be desired. I hope I've gotten it right.)

As we wrote this book together, every so often, I questioned Our Lady's methods. I could see that each and every lesson had great merit in it of itself, but I was a wee bit curious as to why she put them in the order in which she did, and how she came to pick the topics. And, truthfully, my questions were also a ploy to get her to stop dictating for at least a minute, as my hand was cramping here and there.

She told me that I was not to question why. "Just get the Motivational Musings, Righteous Recipes, Pious Projects, Weighty Confessions, Sacred Assignments, faToids, Tasty Tidbits, and Prickly Prayers down on paper, please," she said softly and sweetly as she whacked my forehead with a celery stick.

What strange language, I thought. "Prickly Prayers?" Nevertheless, I learned my lesson. My role is not to question. I have faith that it will all make sense in the end.

Without further ado . . . from Our Lady of Weight Loss to you. Forty-two lessons meant to motivate, inspire, and spur you into action! (I think forty-two may have something to do with the I Ching. I'm still trying to crack her code!)

Think of them as your "kicks in the tush." After all, who couldn't use a good kick in the tush?

The Official Guide to the Virtuous Vocabulary of Our Lady of Weight Loss, aka

THE GLOSSARY

Our Lady of Weight Loss   **the Patron Saint of Permanent Fat Removal.** Our Lady is here to travel the rocky road to Svelteville with you. Statistics show that if you have support you are much more likely to be a successful loser. Buddy up with Our Lady of Weight Loss!

Weight-Loss Artist   **someone who makes art about food instead of eating it and loses weight in the process.** (Janice Taylor invented the profession under the guidance of Our Lady of Weight Loss.)

Weight-Loss Art   **art that is made by a weight-loss artist.** If a picture is worth a thousand words, then a piece of weight-loss art is worth a thousand prayers and pounds permanently removed.

Motivational Musing   *a dish full of useful information.* Sure to enlighten, inspire, and delight.

Tasty Tidbit   *a side dish of fascinating information.*

faToid   *just a dash of fat trivia.*

Righteous Recipe   *a sacri-licious, light mixture of Our Lady of Weight Loss—approved ingredients.* These delicious and healthy recipes were created by an everyday cook, not a gourmet chef. They're idiot-proof and guilt-free. Easy for any dieter to enjoy.

Pious Project   *a D.I.Y. (Do-It-Yourself) arts and crafts project specifically designed to keep your hands and mind occupied for at least two hours!* That's two hours out of the kitchen fruitfully reinforcing the new you.

> The Non-Piggy Bank is one of Our Lady's favorites. Every time you say "No, thank you" to food, you pay yourself! When your Non-Piggy Bank is full, you go on a nonfood shopping spree!

Sacred Assignment   *thought-provoking assignments* that are sure to set your mind into action and jolt your body into fat-melting mode.

Weighty Confessions   *who doesn't fall from grace in the face of chocolate or my favorite food group, fried?* Our Lady provides you an opportunity to confess and move on. You'll feel lighter for it.

I bought my son four packages of Marshmallow Peeps, those cute little chicks that are covered with sugar. You either love them or hate them. Unfortunately, I love them. My son can afford to eat them. I can't. I do buy them for him and I put them in his bedroom. Out of sight, out of mind. Yeah, right! Somehow they're missing this morning.

Prickly Prayer **prayer helps and heals.** Our Lady of Weight Loss is listening.

Kick in the Tush Club **Our Lady's club** for those lighthearted, low-cal-loving, nutrition-friendly folks who crave mammoth portions of food facts, recipes, art, and inspiration.

KICK chapter in Our Lady's book deriving from the Latin word "kick in the tuckus," something we all need from time to time.

Prickly Prayer

Dear Our Lady of Weight Loss,

Please may I thirst for water
and experience with every sip
its miraculous cleansing powers.

May my sins as well as fat be washed away
and permanently eliminated from my body.

And, please,
may there always be a clean bathroom nearby!

Amen.

Kick in the Tush Club Member Oath

Yes, I, _____, need a kick in the tush
and pledge that I will do my best

> to courageously stare down full-fat ice cream;
>
> to remain strong in the face of devil's food cake;
>
> to be responsible for what I put in my mouth;
>
> to respect others' decisions to eat waffles and fries
>   while I just say no;
>
> to use my daily allotment of calories wisely;
>
> to substitute arts and crafts for food whenever
>   appropriate;
>
> to make macaroni necklaces from those nifty
>   mac and cheese kits;
>
> to make the world a better place by setting a
>   healthy example;
>
> and by being a kind Kick in
>   the Tush Club member to all!

Signed: _____

Date: _____

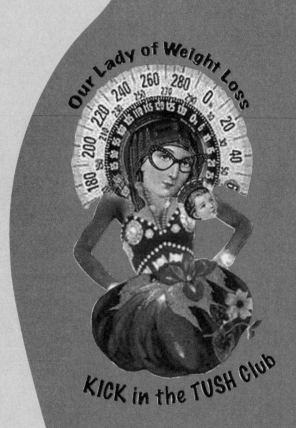

Prickly Prayer

Dear Our Lady of Weight Loss,

As I embark on this weight-loss journey,
I pray that the road ahead is a light one,
Filled with a multitude of tasty low-cal, low-fat desserts.

May my resolve remain strong, my focus steady, and
May the pounds melt away with ease.

Amen.

Our Lady of Cleanliness Is Next to Weightlessness

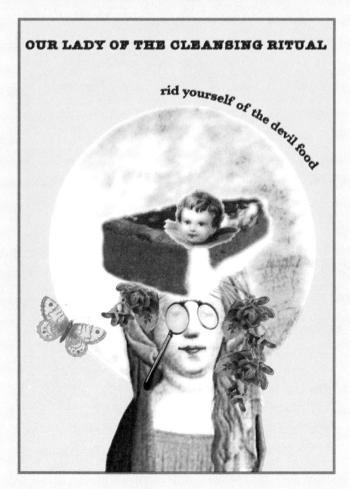

OUR LADY OF THE CLEANSING RITUAL

rid yourself of the devil food

"It's hard to be funny when you have to be clean."

~Mae West

MOTIVATIONAL MUSING
A Cleansing Ritual

The ritual of cleansing is an important aspect of weight loss. Before we can move toward realizing and fully embracing our new selves, we need to break free of those foods to which we have given so much power.

What might they be?

- 100 percent fat-filled ice cream
- 100 percent sugar-filled, fat-filled cake and cookies
- soda
- deep-fried anything (No, fried is not a food group.)
- Cheese Doodles, potato chips, pork rinds

(Your list might be slightly different than mine, but you get the idea.)

- peanut butter

We want to begin anew with balanced and harmonized foods (to be discussed later). But first, let the cleansing begin!

 Dear Our Lady of Weight Loss,

I am miserable. I want to lose weight, but I am completely out of control. I can't seem to get past the idea that the journey I have ahead of me is an unbearably

long and arduous one. I am defeated before I begin. Please help.
~Defeated in Nashville

Dear Defeated,

I know just how you feel. Figuring out a new way of being/eating is exhausting. First things first. You've got to set your intention and commit to yourself. The best way to do this is to perform a ritual, and I know no better ritual than the cleansing ritual. Not only does the cleansing ritual present a fun way to begin your weight-loss journey, but your refrigerator gets clean at the same time! Hang in there. We're going to get you started. You'll have tons of fun and lose weight at the same time! ~Our Lady of Weight Loss

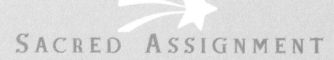

SACRED ASSIGNMENT
The Cleansing Ritual

To begin our cleansing, you will need the following:

1. two cartons
2. Magic Marker (to write on cartons)
3. vinegar
4. baking soda
5. clear ammonia
6. spray bottle
7. sponge

8. bowl
9. a great picture of Our Lady of Weight Loss
10. strength, determination, and resolve

Now . . . follow these easy instructions:

1. Tape an Our Lady image to the front of your cabinet and/or refrigerator. You're going to need a lot of support. Tossing out three-week-old, half-eaten cake is a difficult thing to do.

> Note: There's an Our Lady of Weight Loss cutout doll on page 251 of this book!

2. Empty your cabinets and refrigerator.
3. Separate items into three categories:
   a. foods that you are actually keeping (ketchup and lettuce)
   b. non–Our Lady–approved foods from the pantry, to include Cheese Doodles, creamed corn, scalloped potato mix, Ring Dings, Devil Dogs—the ridiculously high sugar and fat and chemical-laden foods! (Note: If you find a box of mac and cheese, set it aside! You'll use it later for something special.)
   c. foods from the refrigerator that we are just going to dump in the garbage (the cream sauces, leftover cake—whether it is moldy or not).
4. Take the Magic Marker and boldly, with intention and consciousness, write "garbage" on one of the cartons and "donations" on the other.

5. Put non–Our Lady of Weight Loss–approved canned and boxed goods into the donation box.
6. Put half-eaten, nonapproved refrigerator foods into the garbage box and quickly take them to the Dumpster. No last-minute bites!
7. As you rid yourself of the cake, ice cream, candy, heavy bread, butters, bad oils, and Twinkies (by either tossing or donating), be sure to sing the following to the tune of Bob Dylan's "The Times They Are A-Changin.'"

> *Come gather 'round fat cells,*
> *wherever you hide,*
> *and admit that the waters*
> *are flushing you bye!*
> *Accept that it's over*
> *and time for you to fly.*
> *For the scales, they are a-changin'.*

Sing it loud and proud, whether you believe it yet or not!

8. After you're done cleaning and putting the lettuce back in the fridge, you can deliver the donation box to your local church or homeless shelter. Our Lady would really like it if you wrote "Donated in the Name of Our Lady of Weight Loss" on the box.

Now, it's time to clean.

9. Mix together one gallon of hot water, one cup of clear ammonia, a half cup of vinegar, and a quarter cup of baking soda. Pour into a spray bottle, or use from a bowl with a sponge.
10. Clean your refrigerator and cabinets.

11. Once all has been cleaned, burn an Our Lady of Weight Loss candle (or one that has significant meaning to you), and say the following:

Dear Our Lady of Weight Loss,

May my commitment to myself shine as brightly
as my sparkling clean fridge.
May I remember that it is not about willpower.
There is no such thing.
This is about want power.
May I give myself everything I want and deserve.

Amen.

12. Put the rest of the food back in your clean cabinets and refrigerator.
13. Congratulate yourself. You're on your way!

Before you head out to restock your refrigerator with the right stuff, have lunch! Never go food shopping on an empty stomach.

Tasty Tidbit **Cleaning Tips**

♦ To prevent grease and odor buildup on top of the stove after you have cleaned it, simply buff a bit of car wax onto the surface.

♦ Toothpaste contains a gentle abrasive. A little on a soft toothbrush will remove tough stains from countertops!

♦ Get those old pantyhose out and cover a long stick with them (maybe the broom upside down). Run under the refrigerator and on the side of the stove. Get those hard to reach dust bunnies outta there!

♦ Need a quick fix for odors? Dampen a couple of cotton balls with vanilla, almond, or orange extract — or with any pleasing scent — and place them in a shallow dish in your fridge.

♦ The miracle of the brown paper bag! Crumple it up, place it in your veggie bin, and wait forty-eight hours. Odors will be gone, absorbed into the brown.

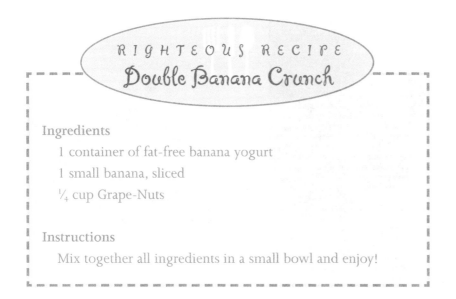

RIGHTEOUS RECIPE
Double Banana Crunch

Ingredients

1 container of fat-free banana yogurt

1 small banana, sliced

¼ cup Grape-Nuts

Instructions

Mix together all ingredients in a small bowl and enjoy!

Nutrition Facts

Serving Size (263g)
Servings Per Container 1

Amount Per Serving

Calories 270   Calories from Fat 5

	% Daily Value*
Total Fat 1g	2%
Saturated Fat 0g	0%
Trans Fat 0g	
Cholesterol 5mg	2%
Sodium 250mg	10%
Total Carbohydrate 59g	20%
Dietary Fiber 5g	20%
Sugars 26g	
Protein 9g	

Vitamin A 20% • Vitamin C 10%

Calcium 20% • Iron 45%

*Percent Daily Values are based on a 2,000 calorie diet. Your daily values may be higher or lower depending on your calorie needs:

	Calories	2,000	2,500
Total Fat	Less Than	65g	80g
Saturated Fat	Less Than	20g	25g
Cholesterol	Less Than	300mg	300 mg
Sodium	Less Than	2,400mg	2,400mg
Total Carbohydrate		300g	375g
Dietary Fiber		25g	30g

Calories per gram:
Fat 9 • Carbohydrate 4 • Protein 4

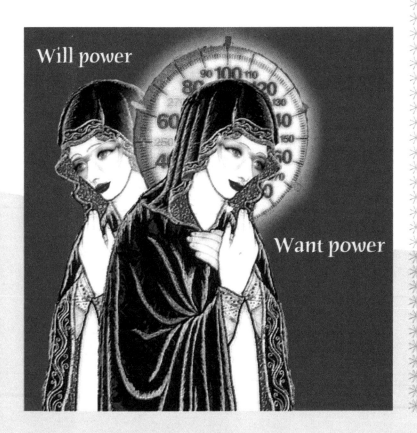

Will power

Want power

Dear Our Lady of Weight Loss,

I must confess the drama that went on in my home last night. (Yes, it was of my own making, but drama nonetheless.)

After completing the cleansing ritual, taking my "donations in the name of Our Lady of Weight Loss" to my local church, after changing the kitty litter, prepping for the next morning, and brushing my teeth, I decided to put out one last fire before going to bed.

I went to put away the paper towels that I had bought two days before. I opened the pantry door and moved a few things to make room for them . . . when I saw it.

There it was peeking out from behind the couscous and whole wheat pasta (all Our Lady—approved, by the way)—a small but deadly 16 ounce jar of super chunk peanut butter.

I froze! How on earth did it survive the pantry purging, the cleansing ritual? Who put it there?

Then I realized. Our Lady of *Weight Loss* was testing me. She was bringing out the big guns!

I told myself to just back away. Close the pantry door; go to bed. It was 11:48 P.M.

At 12:22 A.M., I found myself thinking about a toasted English muffin slathered with peanut butter and sliced bananas.

At 12:53 A.M., I was trying to figure out just how much of that jar I could eat if I didn't eat anything else for the next thirty-six hours.

At 1:27 A.M., I jumped out of bed and made a beeline to my junk drawer.

Where was it? Where was the one thing I needed to save myself from this temptation?

Things were flying out of that drawer willy-nilly. (I found a lost earring, a pair of nail clippers, and a dry cleaning receipt from two years ago).

Then I found it! With my salvation in hand, I yanked open the pantry door, grabbed that jar of PB, and superglued the lid on within an inch of its life.

There you have it. No willpower, but plenty of want power! ~ Leslie McIntosh

Pious Project

OUR LADY OF WEIGHT LOSS'S MAC AND LOW-FAT CHEESE ALTAR

When I cleaned out my pantry at Our Lady's request, I found several boxes of macaroni and cheese hiding behind a rancid bag of Cheese Doodles (which I immediately tossed).

I held the box in my hand, thinking "to cook or not to cook" and—eureka—next thing I knew, I was cutting, pasting, and gluing. Macaroni

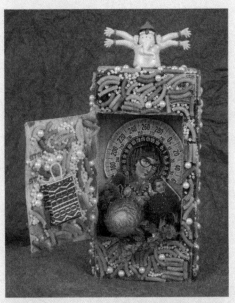

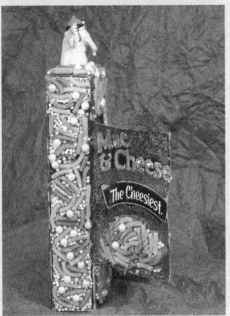

"pearls," "diamonds" . . . Wow! An altar to Our Lady of Weight Loss magically and mysteriously appeared.

It's important to have an altar to Our Lady of Weight Loss in the kitchen. After all, the kitchen is her domain. You better make one too. She'll keep you in line!

SUPPLIES

1 box of mac and cheese your choice of shape
flat razor blade or razor knife
a glue gun or craft glue
glitter glue pens
macaroni "pearls" and "diamonds"
a picture of Our Lady of Weight Loss

INSTRUCTIONS

Leave the top and bottom of the box intact.

Take the blade and cut a door in the front of the box, leaving about an inch on the top, side, and bottom.

Empty contents of box.

Heat up your glue gun and gently glue the macaroni and trim to the box. If you use glitter glue, the macaroni sticks to it, and it's all glittery. What could be better?

Macaroni and Cheese

*E*veryone loves this blue plate special—macaroni and cheese!!!
Serve with a huge leafy green salad, red pepper, and tomatoes.

Note: I made this mac and cheese for some hard-core comfort-
food aficionados, and they *loved* it! In fact, they said it was the *best*
mac and cheese they had ever had. No kidding!

Ingredients

nonfat cooking spray
1 16-oz. container low-fat sour cream
1 8-oz. container low-fat cottage cheese
1 16-oz. box of elbow macaroni, cooked
2 cups low-fat cheese, grated
$\frac{1}{2}$ cup evaporated skim milk
$\frac{1}{4}$ cup green onion, finely chopped
2 eggs
salt and pepper to taste
$\frac{1}{4}$ cup bread crumbs
paprika

Nutrition Facts

Serving Size (162g)
Servings Per Container 8

Amount Per Serving

Calories 360   Calories from Fat 80

	% Daily Value*
Total Fat 9g	**14%**
Saturated Fat 4.5g	**23%**
Trans Fat 0g	
Cholesterol 85mg	**28%**
Sodium 270mg	**11%**
Total Carbohydrate 51g	**17%**
Dietary Fiber 2g	**8%**
Sugars 5g	
Protein 19g	

Vitamin A 10%	•	Vitamin C 2%
Calcium 20%	•	Iron 15%

*Percent Daily Values are based on a 2,000 calorie diet. Your daily values may be higher or lower depending on your calorie needs:

	Calories	2,000	2,500
Total Fat	Less Than	65g	80g
Saturated Fat	Less Than	20g	25g
Cholesterol	Less Than	300mg	300 mg
Sodium	Less Than	2,400mg	2,400mg
Total Carbohydrate		300g	375g
Dietary Fiber		25g	30g

Calories per gram:
Fat 9 • Carbohydrate 4 • Protein 4

Directions

Preheat oven to 350°.

Spray a casserole dish with cooking spray and set aside.

In a blender, mix together sour cream and cottage cheese until smooth.

Combine blended mixture with cooked macaroni, cheese, milk, chopped onion, and eggs (slightly beaten).

Mix well and add salt and pepper to taste.

Pour into prepared casserole dish and sprinkle with bread crumbs and paprika.

Bake covered for 35 minutes, uncover and bake 5 minutes or so more until brown. Everyone's oven is different.

Kick No. 2

Our Lady of the Third Eye

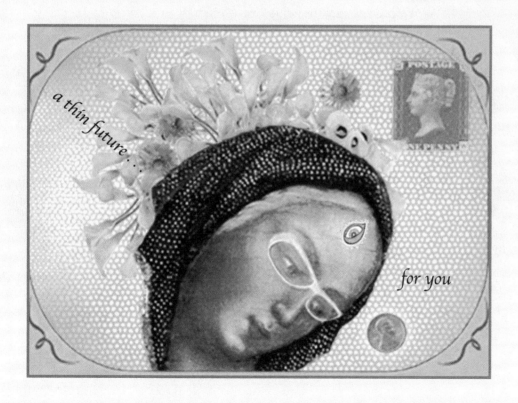

a thin future....

for you

"You create your
opportunities by
asking for them."
~Shakti Gawain

MOTIVATIONAL MUSING
Seeing Is Believing:
The Power of Visualization

Being able to visualize or "see" yourself "thin" is an essential element of permanent fat removal.

Whether we are aware of it or not, we visualize every day. As we process our thoughts, we project them as pictures onto the screens of our mind. Daydreaming, fantasizing, and mental rehearsals are examples of visualization.

Many of us dream of having a new job, going on a hike in the woods, swimming in the warm waters of the Caribbean—all pleasant thoughts and images.

There are times, however, that we get caught in the negative web of mentally reviewing and rehearsing our fears. Have you had a mental fight? Or imagined the unimaginable—gaining back the ten pounds that you just lost? (*Such dark thoughts! Oh my.*)

Many of us don't realize the power of our minds. If you imagine the negative, you will create negativity in your life.

Visualization helps us realize our dreams. When an idea becomes "fixed" in our subconscious, we automatically make decisions that help us move toward it. Athletes are known to utilize visualization to reach their goals. They see themselves performing the perfect dive off the high board, scoring a 10!

According to the book *The Einstein Factor* by Win Wenger and Richard Poe, visualization helps to increase our intelligence. It helps to build the connectors between the neurons in our brains. It's like building a mental muscle. Albert Einstein conducted most of his experiments in his brain—by visualizing them.

Our outside world—what we consider reality—manifests from our mental world. First comes the thought. And from thought, we create our reality.

For those of us who want to remove excess weight permanently it is imperative that we spend a period of time, daily, consciously seeing and creating our new selves.

SACRED ASSIGNMENT
Creative Visualization 101

Here's the skinny on how to create in your mind. Remember, your capacity to visualize grows with practice. So, if your first visualization is short and fuzzy, just give it time to take form.

First, find a quiet place far from the madding crowd. No distractions, please. Get comfortable and relax. Take in a number of slow, deep breaths (see Our Lady of the Deep Cleansing Breath, page 117).

Release the tension of the day, your concerns, and your anxieties with each exhale.

I like to start my visualization as if it's the start of a movie. The clapper guy snaps the clapboard and bellows, "Take one. Our Lady of Weight Loss, the Movie, starring Julia Roberts as Our Lady." Or Meg Ryan—or Jennifer Tilly; I like her voice. Or Halle Barry in her Catwoman suit. Depends on my mood.

Before you start, take in a few more deep, cleansing breaths. (Breathe in; breathe out.) Let your visualization begin. Bring as much detail to your vision as possible. Imagine what you're wearing, your hairstyle, who's with you, the colors, the words, the sounds, the smells, and most importantly, how you feel. Are you comfortable in your new thin body? The more vivid the visualization, the more real it will feel to you, and the more likely it will take form.

Enjoy your visualization.

Dear Our Lady of Weight Loss,

Last night, in those sweet moments just before drifting off to sleep, I visualized that all of my fat was melting off me (like the Wicked Witch of the West) into a puddle at my feet. I was wearing a magical invisible body armor that protected me from the devil's temptations. I stepped out of the puddle and felt lighter than air. I am going to use this dream as my official visualization. Every so often, I'm going to close my eyes and imagine and feel the fat just drippin' off me. . . . Cheers. ~Lighter than Air

Dear Lighter than Air,

What a great visualization—I just love it. Now be careful that people don't slip, slide, and fall in that trail of melted fat! ~Our Lady of Weight Loss

Pious Project

The fortunes from fortune cookies are too good to resist. They are filled with such wonderfully hopeful and uplifting sayings, like "You will be successful in all you do." Wow!

I collect my fortunes. Sometimes I use them for greeting cards, postcards, or bookmarks, but this time I made a fortune cookie frame!

SUPPLIES

1" sponge brushes (You may as well buy at least a dozen. They're great. You can wash them out or throw them out after using them.)

acrylic paint—any bright color (I used an orange/red)

1 wooden picture frame

craft paste

rice paper

fortunes from fortune cookies

pearls, diamonds, little babies, assorted junk!

INSTRUCTIONS

Using one of those fab sponge brushes, give your wooden frame a coat or two of orange and/or red paint. Then rip up some rice paper into bite-size pieces. Dip one of your sponge brushes into the craft paste, and glue down the rice paper, putting craft paste under and over the paper. Rice paper has a great transparency to it. It "melts" into the frame and over your work, giving an illusion of layers. Then paste the fortunes down, any which way. "Controlled chaos" is my m.o. Another layer of rice paper. More fortunes.

Then top it off with a little of this and a little of that. I found an old spoon and toy babies in my box of odds 'n' ends. Perfecto!

Side Bar: One fortune cookie is 28 calories.

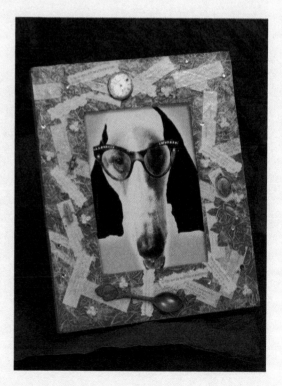

Kick No. 3

Our Lady of the Good Morning Meal

"Once a woman has forgiven her man, she must not reheat his sins for breakfast."
~Marlene Dietrich

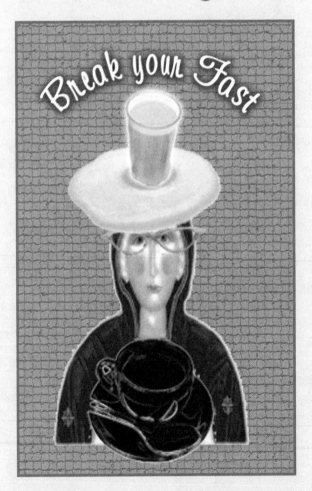

MOTIVATIONAL MUSING
Break Your Fast!

faToid
Breakfast eaters are more likely to look after their health and less likely to catch a cold.

Want to burn calories faster? Eat breakfast! Approximately three thousand men and women who had lost thirty pounds or more and kept it off for at least one year were surveyed by the University of Colorado Health Sciences Department. Do you know what the one common denominator was that these successful losers had in common? You guessed it! They all ate breakfast.

Some people think that skipping breakfast will aid in their weight-loss efforts. Not true! Your metabolism slows down when you sleep. Come morning, you want to get your engines revved up and going as soon as possible. Therefore, the sooner you eat breakfast, the better!

In addition to getting your metabolism burning bright, a recent study conducted at the University of Texas at El Paso found that those who ate a morning meal actually ingested fewer calories over the course of the day.

Skipping meals leads to a state called overhungry, which makes you lose control of your eating because it is more difficult to tell when you are full. If you skip breakfast, you will more than likely more than make up for those calories later in the day.

Eating breakfast also improves concentration, problem-solving ability, mental performance, memory, and mood. Life is tough enough without adding these problems.

Eat up, eat healthy!

Nutrition Facts

Serving Size (126g)
Servings Per Container 4

Amount Per Serving

Calories 130   Calories from Fat 25

	% Daily Value*
Total Fat 3g	**5%**
Saturated Fat 2g	**10%**
Trans Fat 0g	
Cholesterol 10mg	**3%**
Sodium 100mg	**4%**
Total Carbohydrate 24g	**8%**
Dietary Fiber 3g	**12%**
Sugars 16g	
Protein 3g	

Vitamin A 4%	•	Vitamin C 60%
Calcium 6%	•	Iron 4%

*Percent Daily Values are based on a 2,000 calorie diet. Your daily values may be higher or lower depending on your calorie needs:

	Calories	2,000	2,500
Total Fat	Less Than	65g	80g
Saturated Fat	Less Than	20g	25g
Cholesterol	Less Than	300mg	300 mg
Sodium	Less Than	2,400mg	2,400mg
Total Carbohydrate		300g	375g
Dietary Fiber		25g	30g

Calories per gram:
Fat 9 • Carbohydrate 4 • Protein 4

R I G H T E O U S   R E C I P E

Enchanted Muffin

(As breakfast or a dessert—it's that good!)

Ingredients

4 light English muffins (100 calories per muffin)

1 tablespoon of lemon zest

juice from ½ fresh lemon

4 Tbs. of light brown sugar or sugar substitute

2 cups of sliced strawberries and/or blueberries (any berry will do)

4 Tbs. of light cream cheese (reduced fat)

Directions

Pop the light English muffin in the toaster.

In a saucepan, over a high heat, mix together lemon zest, lemon juice, and sugar, stirring until the sugar melts and bubbles. About one minute.

Lower the heat a bit; add berries; and stir until they are heated through.

Spread ½ tablespoon of light cream cheese on each slice of toasted English muffin. Top with warm berries. Enjoy. Two open halves per serving.

Dear Our Lady of Weight Loss,

Honest to goodness, I feel hungry. I am sticking to my plan, but it's just not enough food. Fighting these empty feelings is draining. ~Haunted by Hunger

Dear Haunted by Hunger,

We often mistake thirst for hunger, so make sure you are drinking enough (water, decaffeinated tea, club soda). Be sure to eat breakfast and bulk up on vegetables. You used the words "empty feelings" in your letter. Maybe the hunger has to do with some empty feelings, if you get my drift. Something to munch over.
~Our Lady of Weight Loss

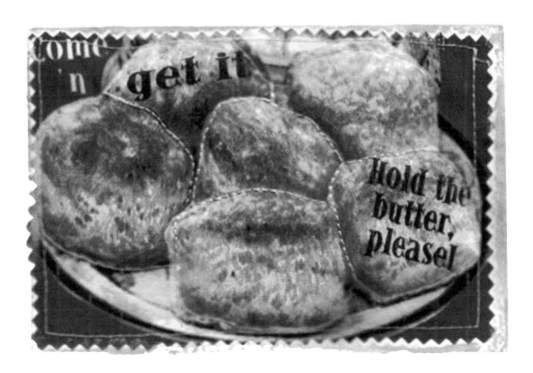

Our Lady of the Evelyn Wood School of Label Reading

"Life isn't about
finding yourself.
Life is about
creating yourself."
~Unknown

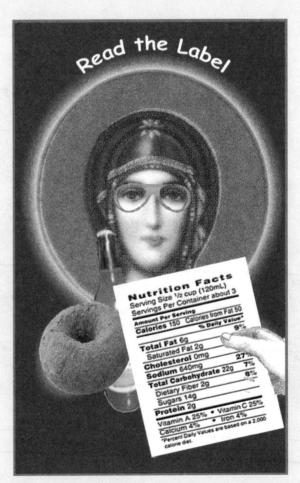

Size Matters!

A deli muffin could weigh in at a ½ pound and contain more than 600 calories. The standard U.S. Department of Agriculture (USDA) 1½ ounce muffin contains approximately 100 calories and is the size of an egg!

*I*n a survey commissioned by the American Institute for Cancer Research, 78 percent of respondents said that eating certain types of food while avoiding others was more important to their weight-loss efforts than eating less food. *Wrong!*

By all means, make healthy choices, but . . . effective weight-loss plans place equal importance on both the kinds and amounts of food ingested. Portion size most certainly matters, because weight loss is based on how many calories you take in and burn off.

What Is a Serving Size?

A "serving" is simply a measure of unit. There is no one definition for a serving size. The food pyramid indicates that an English muffin is two bread servings, but the English muffin box indicates that one muffin is one serving. The standard USDA serving for French fries is about ten (Yikes! I'm in trouble). Would you like to know how many fries are in a Wendy's Great Biggie? About one hundred fries and they weigh in at 530 calories.

How to Get a Handle on Portions?

Weigh and measure first. Invest in measuring spoons, cups, and a food scale. While you're shopping, you might as well pick up a calorie count guidebook and a notebook to keep track honestly of what you put in your mouth! These are great tools for determining portion sizes and calorie counts and are well worth the investment.

Here are some portion (serving) guidelines taken from the USDA food pyramid.

- **Milk, Yogurt, and Cheese**
    - 1 cup of milk or yogurt
    - 1 oz. of natural cheese
    - 2 oz. of processed cheese

- **Meat, Poultry, Dry Beans, Eggs, and Nuts**
    - 2–3 oz. of cooked lean meat, poultry, or fish
    - ½ cup of cooked dry beans
    - 1 egg
    - 2 Tbs. of peanut butter

- **Vegetables**
    - 1 cup of raw leafy vegetables
    - 1 cup of other vegetables, cooked or chopped raw
    - 1 cup of vegetable juice

- **Fruit**
    - 1 medium apple, banana, orange
    - ½ cup of chopped, cooked, or canned fruit (in its natural juices—watch out for added sugar)
    - ½ cup of fruit juice

- **Bread, Cereal, Rice, or Pasta**
    - 1 slice of bread or 1 oz. of bread
    - 1 oz. of ready-to-eat cereal
    - ½ cup of cooked cereal, rice, or pasta

Tasty Tidbit **Talk to the Hand**

When away from home, here are some handy guidelines to keep in mind:

- ♦ Guesstimating Portion Sizes

    3 oz. of meat, poultry, or fish are about the size of a women's palm

    $1/2$ cup of cut fruit, vegetables, or pasta is about the size of a small fist

    1 cup of milk, yogurt, or chopped fresh greens is about the size of a small hand holding a tennis ball

    1 oz. of cheese is about the size of your thumb

    1 tsp. of margarine is about the size of your thumb tip

- ♦ Dining Out

    To limit the amount you eat when dining out, try following some of these strategies:

    Order an appetizer as an entrée (main dish).

    Split an entrée with another person.

    Cut your entrée in half as soon as you get it, and ask your waiter to wrap the other half "to go" ASAP.

    If you're in a fast-food restaurant, never ever utter the words *extra value* or *super size* with meals.

RIGHTEOUS RECIPE
Waldorf Salad à la Our Lady

Ingredients

4 apples, unpeeled, cored and chopped into bite-size pieces
(about 3 cups)

juice from ½ fresh lemon

⅓ cup raisins (plumped*)

⅔ cup chopped celery

¼ cup walnut halves

¼ cup reduced-fat mayonnaise (25 calories per tablespoon)

1 Tbs. sugar

*Plumped:

Place raisins in bowl and add enough warm tap water to cover them. Let them sit for a few minutes, absorbing the water, as they happily and peacefully plump up. After they are sufficiently plump, carefully and with love squeeze out excess water.

Directions

Mix everything together in a medium-size bowl. Let it chill overnight. Something yummy and crunchy to look forward to!

Nutrition Facts

Serving Size (206g)
Servings Per Container 4

Amount Per Serving		
Calories 170	Calories from Fat 60	
		% Daily Value*
Total Fat 7g		**11%**
Saturated Fat 1g		**5%**
Trans Fat 0g		
Cholesterol 0mg		**0%**
Sodium 150mg		**6%**
Total Carbohydrate 29g		**10%**
Dietary Fiber 3g		**12%**
Sugars 4g		
Protein 3g		
Vitamin A 2%	•	Vitamin C 150%
Calcium 2%	•	Iron 4%

*Percent Daily Values are based on a 2,000 calorie diet. Your daily values may be higher or lower depending on your calorie needs:

		Calories	2,000	2,500
Total Fat	Less Than		65g	80g
Saturated Fat	Less Than		20g	25g
Cholesterol	Less Than		300mg	300 mg
Sodium	Less Than		2,400mg	2,400mg
Total Carbohydrate			300g	375g
Dietary Fiber			25g	30g

Calories per gram:
Fat 9 • Carbohydrate 4 • Protein 4

Dear Our Lady of Weight Loss,

I love that you used your creativity to help you lose weight. I am trying to do that. I was wondering if you had to keep food journals, and what is in your pantry? My weakness is also anything cakelike: donuts, cupcakes, and such. I did the whole food journal thing a couple of years ago. It did help for a while, and then I couldn't take it anymore. All I thought about was my food intake. I would like to think about food less, not more. Any advice? Oh, I also have two young children, they are two and a half and six years old. ~Thanks, Shannon B.

Dear Shannon,

My hat's off to anyone who has children and loses weight! I confess that when I would serve my kids, I'd eat the leftovers on my way back into the kitchen. We give food such crazy mind-altering powers. In answer to your question, yes, I did and do keep a food journal. In fact, my suggestion is to make it as lush a food journal as possible. Use glitter, stickers, cutout photos of food; write in different color pens. Make it fun!!!! If you want to write a line or two at the end of the day about what was going on—like a regular diary—do so. When you look back over the weeks and months, you will learn all kinds of cool stuff about yourself. Very insightful! Oh, my pantry is void of cake, cookies, candy, etc. No point in torturing myself! I keep a bowl filled with fresh fruit and tons of vegetables cut and ready to go. ~Our Lady of Weight Loss

Pious Project
THE WEIGHTY BOOKMARK: THE INSPIRATIONAL MESSAGES FROM BEYOND BOOKMARK

One of my favorite pastimes is to "communicate" with Our Lady of Weight Loss. Sometimes she speaks to me through magazines. It's Ouija boardesque. You know, her hand is pushing my hand to cut

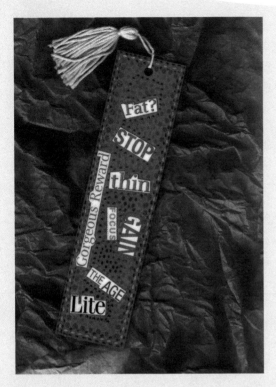

and paste the right words. I am sure, as she has told me, that if you believe, she will "communicate" with you as well.

SUPPLIES

magazines (You can use any publication. I find that either diet magazines or yoga/spiritual magazines are best. They are chock-full of food words and positive phrases.)

scissors

cardboard or oak tag (I'm having an elementary school flashback.) Cut into 2" x 8" pieces

glue stick

hole-punch tassel (optional)

INSTRUCTIONS

Gather your magazines and scissors and sit someplace comfortable, where the feng shui is good and you are feeling open to receiving messages from Our Lady of Weight Loss.

Graze through magazines and rip and/or cut out words and/or phrases that grab you. Whatever you do—*do not think.* Just gather words.

Place words on 2" x 8" cardboard. Use glue stick to adhere to cardboard.

Decorate with opaque paint markers. Dots, swirls, stars! Go wiggy. Cover both sides of cardboard.

Get it laminated. Punch a hole near the top and pull the tassel through and tie.

Prickly Prayer

Dear Our Lady of the Hair Trigger,

May that tired old tape that plays in my head—
the one that triggers me into a mindless pursuit
of chips, chocolate, and other sinner's delights,
be permanently erased!
And replaced by a soft, gentle breeze that whispers
"luscious fruit."

Amen.

Kick No. 5

Our Lady Has a Hair Trigger

"When my time comes, just skin me and put me up there on Trigger, just as though nothing had ever changed."

~Roy Rogers

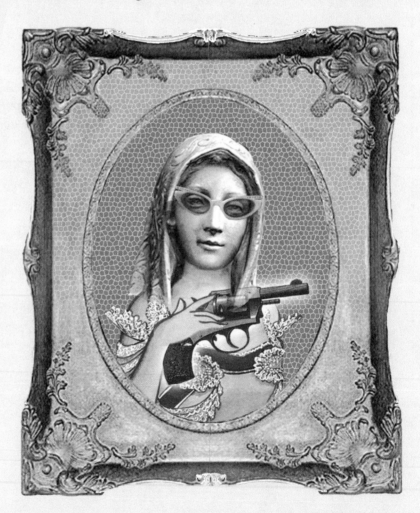

fa T oid

Eating too few carbs can
actually trigger cravings
for more carbs.

MOTIVATIONAL MUSING
Somebody Stop Me, Please!

Trigger foods are foods that get the better of us, that set off some sort of irrational chain reaction that causes us to overeat, binge—go crazy.

Over the course of the day, our brains send out a number of hunger messages. Sometimes we really are hungry. (I experienced that once.) Perhaps you haven't eaten for a number of hours and your stomach is empty.

And then there are the times when the mere mention of fries, or the aroma wafting through the air as we pass the neighborhood bakery, or even a food commercial sets us off.

I have my own set of high-calorie, fat-laden trigger foods that screw up my stopping mechanism. Chocolate cupcakes with fancy icing send me to a place that is diametrically opposed to my weight-loss/health goals.

How to Deal with Trigger Foods?

First, identify your trigger foods. You need to know what you're up against. Now, stay away from them. Do not keep them in the house. (Really, what kind of masochist are you?) Some people tell me that they have children who require these food items. Like a 910 calorie, 64 fat grams, 7 ounce bag of BBQ potato chips? Really? I don't think so.

Replace trigger foods with healthy choices. Instead of potato chips, make baked potato chips. A banana will calm the sweet tooth. Low-fat chocolate pudding is pretty good as well.

Never let yourself get hungry. An empty stomach is a recipe for disaster.

Should you overindulge—trigger yourself into a sugar high—do not freak out. It's not over. Dust off those cookie crumbs and hop back on the Our Lady of Weight Loss bandwagon.

RIGHTEOUS RECIPE
Pleasurable Peaches

Ingredients

½ cup skim milk ricotta cheese (can substitute low-fat cottage cheese)

1 Tbs. confectioners' sugar or sugar substitute (your choice)

4 flour tortillas (10 inch)

1 tsp. butter, melted

2 tsps. cinnamon sugar mixture (mix together 1 tsp. cinnamon; 1 tsp. sugar)

4 peaches, sliced and pitted

Directions

Preheat broiler.

In a small bowl, combine ricotta cheese and confectioners' sugar; set aside.

Arrange tortillas on a broiler pan; brush with butter, sprinkle with cinnamon sugar.

Put sliced peaches in a bowl.

Broil about 6 inches from heat, until they are a nice light brown. Somewhere around three minutes. Watch carefully!

Cool slightly, spread with ricotta, and then place peach slices on top.

WEIGHTY CONFESSION

Forgive Me for I Have Sinned

I don't know what happened—seriously. I had one paper-thin sliver of carrot cake (a vegetable, no less!), and then next thing you know I was, like, off to the races. Bam, pow, rational thinking down the drain. I sit here before you, in a stupor, asking for forgiveness.

All Is Forgiven.

Move On.

Nutrition Facts		
Serving Size (285g)		
Servings Per Container 4		

Amount Per Serving		
Calories 230	Calories from Fat 35	
		% Daily Value*
Total Fat 4g		6%
Saturated Fat 1.5g		8%
Trans Fat 0g		
Cholesterol 5mg		2%
Sodium 290mg		12%
Total Carbohydrate 40g		13%
Dietary Fiber 4g		16%
Sugars 20g		
Protein 13g		

Vitamin A 15%	•	Vitamin C 20%
Calcium 6%	•	Iron 6%

*Percent Daily Values are based on a 2,000 calorie diet. Your daily values may be higher or lower depending on your calorie needs:

	Calories	2,000	2,500
Total Fat	Less Than	65g	80g
Saturated Fat	Less Than	20g	25g
Cholesterol	Less Than	300mg	300 mg
Sodium	Less Than	2,400mg	2,400mg
Total Carbohydrate		300g	375g
Dietary Fiber		25g	30g

Calories per gram:
Fat 9 • Carbohydrate 4 • Protein 4

Kick No. 6

Our Lady Suffers from Constant Cravings

"Desires are
egotistic cravings."
~Shui-ch'ing Tzu

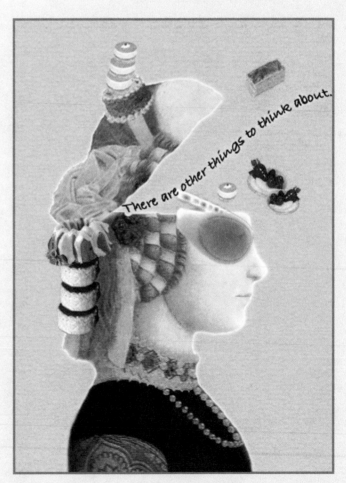

54

Can't Get My Mind Over You

fa T oid

Ninety-seven percent of
women get cravings on
a regular basis.

*a*re you oh so in the mood for something sweet, or maybe something salty, crunchy, creamy? Chocolatey (a category unto itself)? Or fried (my favorite food group)? You're not alone.

According to a study conducted by the University of Calgary in Alberta, Canada, 97 percent of women have experienced food cravings, versus 68 percent of men. Apparently, women are more likely to turn to food than men, as men tend to find other things to do.

Let's be clear. We're talking about cravings—not hunger pangs. And while it may feel as if cravings strike from left field—that is, out of the blue—for no reason, research shows that they show up at the same time of day and get activated by the same reasons over and over again.

So, **let's get hip to our cravings** and meet them head on.

- ➤ **Afternoon delight.** Many experience cravings in the mid-afternoon—somewhere around 3:00 P.M. I call it the "craving not to be at work" syndrome. Our blood glucose levels are in the Dumpsters. If we see or think about food, we're off and running to the vending machine for a bag of chips, or to our friend's heavily-stocked-with-goodies desk down the hall.

- ➤ **The FATS.** There are the cravings that are triggered by emotions. They are called the dreaded FATS (fear, anxiety, tension, stress). We think that if we eat a candy bar, a piece of chocolate cake, or a burger and fries that we will feel better. We may for a short time, as the chocolate is melting in our mouths (not our hands), but in the end, we're more likely to say, "What was I thinking?"

- **SAD.** Then there's SAD (seasonal affective disorder). The winter's diminished sunlight may make us sad and leave us craving carbohydrates in order to lift our serotonin levels and feel better.
- **Memories and associations.** And sometimes cravings are triggered by memory. If you're visiting your great aunt Hilda, and she served the best double chocolate layer cake when you were a kid, seeing her may just trigger a serious need for double chocolate layer cake.

What to do? Prepare and strategize!

- **Remember the "fifteen-minute rule."** If a craving hits, chances are it will pass within fifteen minutes. So sit it out, or walk it out (even better). More often than not, you will have moved past the craving and not given in to the call of the vending machine.
- **Keep healthy snacks** on hand for the midafternoon nosedive.
- **Spicy foods** can satisfy taste buds. Have a spiced-up virgin Mary! (Not a bloody Mary. Hold the alcohol. Save the calories and stay in control.)
- **Clean sweep.** Make sure there are no candy bars hidden in your desk or night table at home.
- **Eat every three hours.** Minimeals help to keep the glucose levels from crashing.
- **Do not skip breakfast.**
- **Plan a healthy lunch and dinner.**
- **Find a friend.** If you're in an emotional twist, seek a friendly ear.

Tasty Tidbit You'll be shocked to learn that the top sweet and salty foods that women crave are chocolate, potato chips, cookies, and French fries.

And here are some alternative choices:

In lieu of chips, try some baked potato fries or 94 percent fat-free potato chips.

Two whole wheat Fig Newtons are about 110 calories. As long as you stick to two, you'll be okay.

RIGHTEOUS RECIPE
Baked Fries

I love French fries and often indulge in baked fries. Here's how you do it. Slice one medium-size potato as thin as you can. Then spray the slices with olive oil Pam and sprinkle with salt. Roast at 400° until golden brown. The thinner the chips, the faster they cook.

Nutrition Facts	
Serving Size (173g)	
Servings Per Container 1	

Amount Per Serving	
Calories 160	Calories from Fat 0

	% Daily Value*
Total Fat 0g	**0%**
Saturated Fat 0g	**0%**
Trans Fat 0g	
Cholesterol 0mg	**0%**
Sodium 15mg	**1%**
Total Carbohydrate 36g	**12%**
Dietary Fiber 4g	**16%**
Sugars 2g	
Protein 4g	

Vitamin A 0%	•	Vitamin C 30%	
Calcium 2%	•	Iron 10%	

*Percent Daily Values are based on a 2,000 calorie diet. Your daily values may be higher or lower depending on your calorie needs:

		Calories	2,000	2,500
Total Fat	Less Than		65g	80g
Saturated Fat	Less Than		20g	25g
Cholesterol	Less Than		300mg	300 mg
Sodium	Less Than		2,400mg	2,400mg
Total Carbohydrate			300g	375g
Dietary Fiber			25g	30g

Calories per gram:
Fat 9 • Carbohydrate 4 • Protein 4

OUR LADY SUFFERS FROM CONSTANT CRAVINGS   57

Dear Our Lady of Weight Loss,

I quit smoking. I stopped eating meat cold turkey! But I just can't seem to get a handle on sugar. I've got a sugar Jones bigger than Bugs Bunny's front teeth. What can I do? ~Sweet Sally

Dear Sweet Sally,

Other than substituting fruit for candy and baked chips for fries, you may want to consider meditation or breathing techniques. Sometimes we eat because we're stressed to the nines, and meditation, breathing, and taking long walks can help to reduce the chronic stress that may underlie your cravings. No one said it would be easy, but it's worth it. ~Our Lady of Weight Loss

Pious Project
LET ME BE LIGHT

I was shopping—burning up calories left and right as I motored through the aisles at my favorite department store—when I came upon this bare lamp that was screaming for some embellishment. My inner bulb went off—"Let Me Be Light."

I quickly purchased her, headed home, and in no time had this cool lamp for my studio.

Here's the funny thing: I've never been very good at following instructions. After I'd finished gluing, pasting, and sewing the fringe, trim, and real dried green peas onto the shade, I realized that I had positioned the shade upside down. It was too late to turn it over. Fringe has to dangle. But as it turned out, it was a happy accident if ever there was one. I love the way the lightbulb sticks out of the top. From now on, it's upside down for me!

SUPPLIES

double-sided tape	needle and invisible thread
1 lamp shade	green peas
tassel/fringe	glitter glue
lace	cement glue
printed words	

INSTRUCTIONS

Run a thin line of double-sided tape along the top and bottom rims of the lamp shade. This will hold your tassel and lace in place.

Then run your tassel trim on the bottom and your lace trim on the top.

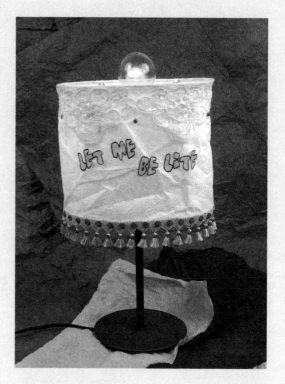

Think of words that inspire or thumb through a magazine until something grabs you. Either type them and print (nice and neat), write them on paper (fancy and scroll), or cut from a magazine. Using a little piece of double-sided tape on each word, gently place and press them onto the lamp shade—just enough to hold them in place while you sew them on with your needle and invisible thread.

Dab a little glitter glue on the round side of the green pea.

When it's dry, place a tiny dab of cement glue on the flat side of the green pea. Gently place onto shade (as seen in photo).

You're free to embellish your shade any way you like. Try buttons, faux fur, beads, glitter. Whatever lights your light!

Kick No. 7

Our Lady of the Plaque-Free Smile

"Start every day with a smile and get it over with."

~W. C. Fields

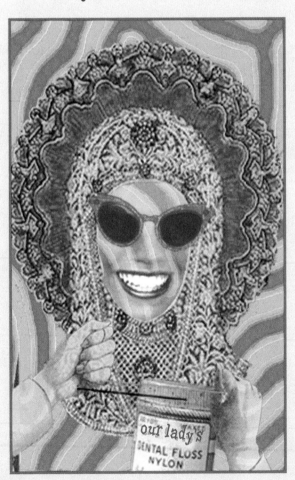

MOTIVATIONAL MUSING
Plaque-Free

Flossing and brushing promotes weight loss. Taste and food particles linger in your mouth and can trigger the desire to eat. If you can't brush and floss when out, try rinsing with mouthwash. (Keep a small bottle in your bag.) Get in there, clean those teeth, and neutralize your taste buds fast!

There are plenty of other benefits from good dental care.

In fact, one of the key contributing factors to longer life is daily flossing! Researchers aren't quite sure why, but they think it could be that the mouth serves as a gateway to the rest of the body, giving the bacteria in plaque a way in. Or, it could be that people who floss tend to be more health conscious than people who don't.

Flossing is one of the best weapons against tooth decay and gum disease. The benefits are many: cleaner teeth, healthier gums, fresher breath, possibly less arterial plaque, and best of all, in the long run, a smaller tush! Your dentist or hygienist will be happy to demonstrate proper flossing techniques. Flossing is well worth the effort.

faToid

Long before the days of floss, mouthwash, and toothpaste, black teeth were considered trendy, hip, and cool in the Orient. To achieve this (might we call it "Goth") preferred effect, women stained their teeth with black dye made from eggplant. They then polished to a brilliant gleam.

Tasty Tidbit **If you want to make your teeth look whiter (and who doesn't?), try wearing a bright shade of lipstick, like red or pink! Oranges and browns actually draw attention to the stains. (For those — such as me — who don't look good in red or pink lipstick, sorry.)**

WEIGHTY CONFESSION

Forgive Me for I Have Sinned

I feel so dirty. I got home late last night from a volunteer program I assist with, had been gone the entire weekend, and had no food in the house and not enough time to make coffee and be on time for work. So I stopped by McDonald's and got an egg biscuit and—for the first time in as long as I can remember—hash browns. I sullied myself for the sake of convenience and I can feel the sluggish movements of transfats gooping their way through my arteries on their direct passage to my derriere. Ah, well . . . nothing to do but re-create my commitment to my own health and well-being and dance on . . .

All Is Forgiven.
Move On.

R I G H T E O U S   R E C I P E
Homemade
Tooth-Whitening Paste

NOT FOR
CONSUMPTION

1 tsp. baking soda

a few drops of hydrogen peroxide

Mix together and make a paste. Use twice weekly.

(Check with your dentist, first!)

Our Lady of Self-eSTEAM Your Vegetables

"Behold I have given you every herb-bearing seed upon the earth, and all the trees that have in themselves seed of their own kind, to be your meat."

~Genesis 1:29

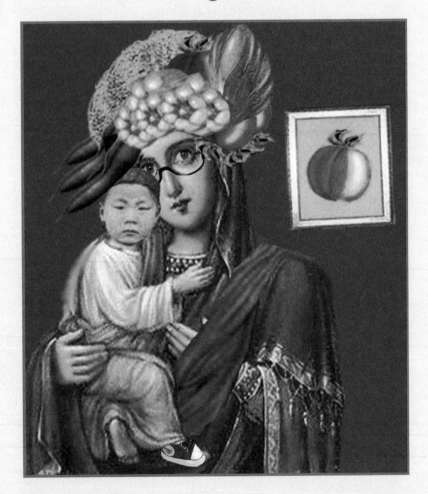

fa T oid

There is no clear
botanical distinction
between vegetables and
fruits. Most vegetables
consist largely of water,
making them lower in
calories than fruit.

MOTIVATIONAL MUSING

Stop!
Don't Throw Those Veggies out
with the Bath Water!

Do you suffer from **lachanophobia**? Each year "fear of vegetables" causes countless people needless distress. This phobia may be due to the fact that for years you have been ingesting overboiled, mushy mounds of bland vegetables that have left you frozen in a field of tasteless greens.

Did you know that the longer you cook vegetables, the more vitamins and nutritional value is lost? The best way to retain their color, flavor, texture, and nutrients is to steam 'em and serve 'em up fast.

Here's what researchers who published their findings in the *Journal of the Science of Food and Agriculture* found:

- **Microwaving** vegetables killed 74 percent to 97 percent of the antioxidant compounds that reduce the risk of lung cancer and heart disease.
- **Boiling** eradicated 66 percent of their flavonoids.
- **Blanching** (briefly submerging vegetables in boiling water) before freezing caused them to lose up to 33 percent of their vitamin C content and more than 50 percent of their folic acid.

But **steaming** caused only a minimal loss, 10 percent, of antioxidants. Why? Because the vegetable isn't in direct contact with water, so there's no direct leaching of antioxidants.

If vegetables are at the bottom of your favorite food list, perhaps you are just plain bored with the same ol'. Make a conscious effort to try something new. How about artichokes, bok choy, leeks, pea pods, eggplant, zucchini?

Nutrition Facts

Serving Size (171g)
Servings Per Container 4

Amount Per Serving

Calories 60	Calories from Fat 5

	% Daily Value*
Total Fat 0.5g	1%
Saturated Fat 0g	0%
Trans Fat 0g	
Cholesterol 0mg	0%
Sodium 280mg	12%
Total Carbohydrate 12g	4%
Dietary Fiber 4g	16%
Sugars 3g	
Protein 4g	

Vitamin A 20%	•	Vitamin C 230%
Calcium 8%	•	Iron 8%

*Percent Daily Values are based on a 2,000 calorie diet. Your daily values may be higher or lower depending on your calorie needs:

	Calories	2,000	2,500
Total Fat	Less Than	65g	80g
Saturated Fat	Less Than	20g	25g
Cholesterol	Less Than	300mg	300 mg
Sodium	Less Than	2,400mg	2,400mg
Total Carbohydrate		300g	375g
Dietary Fiber		25g	30g

Calories per gram:
Fat 9 • Carbohydrate 4 • Protein 4

RIGHTEOUS RECIPE
Blessed Broccoli

Steam a head or two of broccoli with:

Ingredients
lemon herb pepper
¼ cup white wine vinegar (such as white wine fig—my new favorite)
2 Tbs. chopped fresh thyme
fresh ground pepper to taste

Directions
Steam broccoli. Toss all ingredients together.
There are so many great vinegars to choose from. You can't go wrong.

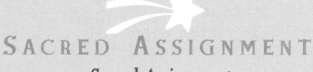

SACRED ASSIGNMENT
Sacred Assignment

Self-*esteam* YourSelf. While you're busy steaming your vegetables, how about some positive self-esteem talk?

Be sure to compliment yourself at least three times a day!

"I love my NuYawk accent."

"Look at me—steaming my vegetables! I'm so great."

"I'm a good person. I listened to my sister complain about her kid's nanny, and I didn't say one word!"

WEIGHTY CONFESSION
Forgive Me for I Have Sinned

I could see the neon light blinking H O T from my dorm room. What was I to do? Cramming for exams, no real food for days (okay, hours). I could not resist. I went out on a Krispy Kreme crumb run. I devoured a baker's dozen.

All Is Forgiven.
Move On.

Kick No. 9

Our Lady Worships the Sun

"To love and be loved is to feel the sun from both sides."
~ David Viscott

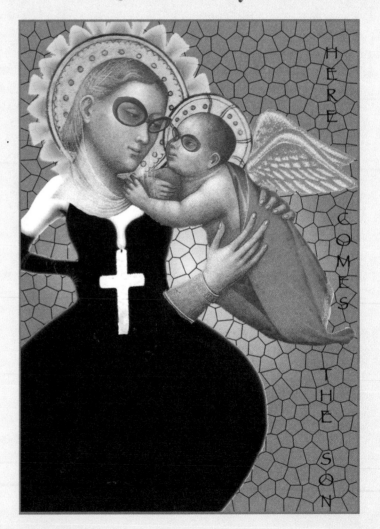

MOTIVATIONAL MUSING
Here Comes the Sun

faToid

The sun is a big ball of
gases, and it gives off
energy in the form of
light and heat.

The Sun represents power, glory, illumination, vitality, and life force.

It's no wonder that too little of it can activate cravings for fatty, high-calorie foods like cakes, cookies, and chips. Lack of sunlight reduces the brain's production of serotonin, the mood-boosting brain chemical that not only helps us feel happy but also suppresses food cravings and bingeing.

Kick those dreary blues away; ward off cravings and bingeing. Walk on the sunny side of the street! Open your drapes and blinds. If you work in a windowless office, take a power walk at lunchtime. Twenty minutes of sunlight a day should do it. However, you must remember to put on your sunscreen lotion and a hat.

Most sun damage occurs within the first ten to twenty minutes of exposure. So, if you think you don't need to put on your SPF (sun protection factor) lotion before picking up your mail, you are mistaken. The paler your skin, the less melanin it has for absorbing UV rays. Doctors recommend that you put on your sunscreen at least twenty minutes before you go outside.

Tasty Tidbit **Using sunscreen and protecting ourselves from the sun could prevent up to 80 percent of skin cancers.**

Dear Our Lady of Weight Loss,

I understand that overexposure to the sun causes sunburn, wrinkles, freckles, skin texture changes, dilated blood vessels, and skin cancers. But I still crave her and long to sit on the beach (for hours and hours) and soak in her rays. I sit pale and sad, in the shade. ~Yours, In Desperate Need of a Tan

Dear In Desperate Need of a Tan,

Ahhh, yes. The rays of the sun do feel good, and a good tan is something that we admire, strive for! How about a compromise? Sit on the beach in the early or late part of the day, after applying sunscreen with a high SPF. Take twenty-minute walks when you can. Those rays are strong, and if you protect yourself, your tanning may be slower and less than that of George Hamilton, but it's the safer, less orange route. ~Our Lady of Weight Loss

RIGHTEOUS RECIPE
Sun-Sational Sun-Dried Dip

Ingredients

2 cups 2% fat cottage cheese

1 small green onion, chopped into small chunks

1 red pepper, chopped

1 yellow pepper, chopped

1 jalapeño pepper, chopped

¼ cup sun-dried tomatoes, chopped

2 Tbs. fresh basil, chopped

2 tsps. lemon juice, from fresh lemon

pepper to taste

Directions

Combine all ingredients in blender; process until smooth, stopping once to scrape sides. Serve with crudités.

Pious Project
FLORAL FANTASY

One day, I was watching *Queer Eye for the Straight Guy*. They said that when going to a friend's home for dinner, we should opt to bring something other than flowers, because when you hand your hostess a bouquet of flowers, she's got to find a vase and arrange them. You've just added another chore to her already long list of hostessy things to do.

Good point. But wait a minute! What if we brought the flowers that were already in a vase? Something the hostess with the mostess could just place on the table? Something colorful and fun.

With this idea in mind, I glittered up an empty spray butter bottle and a couple of small detergent containers. I like that they are obviously no-frills containers. They get a good laugh, they're a great conversation piece, and they sparkle.

I'm ready for another dinner invitation! Somebody—invite me, please.

SUPPLIES

sponge brushes

craft glue

a photo of someone you love, your pet, their pet, an icon. Whatever
   suits you.

glitter glue (gold, blue, green, red)

empty plastic containers

flowers

INSTRUCTIONS

Using a sponge brush and craft glue, paste a photo in the center of
your container and squeeze the glitter glue around it. Do the same on
the backside as well.

Alternatively, follow the colors and patterns of the containers and
"color" with your color glitter glue.
Squeeze it directly out of the bottle.
Yes, it's just like coloring with
crayons, but this time, you only have
to stay in the lines if you want to.

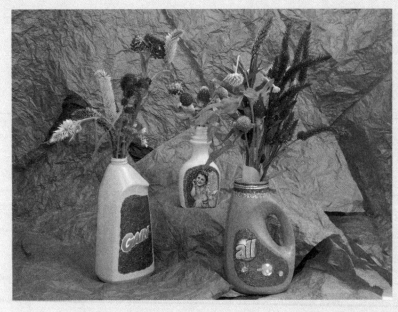

Prickly Prayer

Dear Our Lady of a Dozen Delectable Morsels,

May "the three squares" be transformed
To a half dozen delectable morsels,
Ingested every two hours on the half.
May tasty tidbits swirl through my body,
Leading the mysterious metabolism to
Change its lagging stride
To a run,
to a gold medal win.

Burn swiftly.
Amen.

Our Lady Eats a Dozen Delectable Morsels

"Success to me
is having ten
honeydew melons,
and eating only
the top half of
each one."

~Barbra Streisand

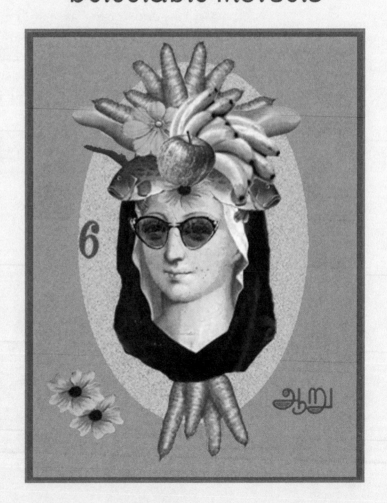

MOTIVATIONAL MUSING
Grazing on a Sunny Afternoon

faᵀoid

New Jersey has more
diners than any other
state and is sometimes
called the diner capital
of the world.

The Meal: Whose idea was it anyway? Did cavemen eat three squares?

Whatever its origin, three meals a day—for me—is a thing of the past. I instinctively tossed major meals out the window at the very start of my weight-loss plan. Since I've been grazing all day, every day, I've stumbled across one article after another touting the incredible benefits of eating six minimeals versus three major meals.

Experts say that eating minimeals:

- decreases the chance of a ravenous hunger setting in and taking over (causing you to act in a reprehensible, hoggish manner);
- helps control cholesterol and blood sugar levels, and thereby can help to prevent heart disease and Type 2 diabetes;
- burns approximately 10 percent more calories a day than eating large meals because it takes calories to burn calories;
- helps the body absorb more nutrients.

Heavy meals make the heart beat up to 30 percent faster, thereby increasing the risk of heart attack. Smaller meals lessen this effect.

Body fat typically doubles between the ages of twenty and sixty. Research shows that older women who eat less but more often burn fat equally as well as younger women who eat three larger meals per day, and those who eat four to six smaller meals per day have less body fat than those eating two or three meals a day, despite the fact that they are eating the same amount of calories.

Eating two to three meals a day, with long stretches between the meals, can potentially trick the body into thinking it is in starvation mode, and actually slow the body down to its resting metabolic rate. So it's not worth bragging, "I barely ate today."

Tasty Tidbit **Minimeal suggestions for those on the run:**
- ♦ a hard-boiled egg or two. (Deviled eggs, if you are feeling fancy!)
- ♦ nonfat yogurt and fruit
- ♦ small bag of baked potato chips
- ♦ low-fat/low-cal soup
- ♦ cucumber and tomato salad (dressing on the side!)
- ♦ a cup of turkey chili

RIGHTEOUS RECIPES
The Devil's Eggs

(Devilishly good, that is!)

Ingredients
1 dozen hard-boiled eggs, preferably free-range and organic
$\frac{1}{3}$ cup reduced-fat mayonnaise
1 sweet pickle, diced
2 heaping Tbs. of honey dijon mustard
juice from 1 fresh lemon
hot sauce, 2 major shakes—3 if you like it spicy

salt and pepper, to taste

fresh parsley, if you have it

Directions

Take hard-boiled eggs and cut the long way. Take yokes out and put in medium-size mixing bowl.

Add reduced-fat (not light) mayonnaise (read the labels: 25 calories per tablespoon versus 50 calories per tablespoon!).

Mix in the rest of the ingredients until smooth and creamy.

Then take a teaspoon of egg mixture and neatly place in the whites. (Try not to lick your fingers too often.)

If you like, you can sprinkle a little paprika on the top. The red looks nice against the yellow.

Nutrition Facts

Serving Size (77g)
Servings Per Container 6

Amount Per Serving

Calories 110   Calories from Fat 70

	% Daily Value*
Total Fat 8g	**12%**
Saturated Fat 2g	**10%**
Trans Fat 0g	
Cholesterol 190mg	**63%**
Sodium 310mg	**13%**
Total Carbohydrate 5g	**2%**
Dietary Fiber 0g	**0%**
Sugars 2g	
Protein 5g	

Vitamin A 4%   •   Vitamin C 10%

Calcium 2%   •   Iron 4%

*Percent Daily Values are based on a 2,000 calorie diet. Your daily values may be higher or lower depending on your calorie needs:

		Calories	2,000	2,500
Total Fat	Less Than		65g	80g
Saturated Fat	Less Than		20g	25g
Cholesterol	Less Than		300mg	300mg
Sodium	Less Than		2,400mg	2,400mg
Total Carbohydrate			300g	375g
Dietary Fiber			25g	30g

Calories per gram:
  Fat 9 • Carbohydrate 4 • Protein 4

WEIGHTY CONFESSION

Forgive Me for I Have Sinned

I had two (count 'em) *large* Bergdorf Blondes (orange juice, milk, half-and-half, sugar, vanilla, and Absolut Citron. Lots of Absolut Citron.), which lowered my resistance to spaghetti and meatballs. And chocolate layer cake for dessert. Glory be. Stepped on the scale this morning with no ill effects. (Thank you for your grace and forgiveness.) Will do better from now on!

All Is Forgiven.
Move On.

Pious Project

TAPE MEASURE BRACELET

If you've got a tape measure lying around the house, and the thought of wrapping it around your waist, hips, or thighs is just too overwhelming, why not make a groovy, funky, fun bracelet out of it?! I wear mine all the time, and it never ceases to amaze and delight!

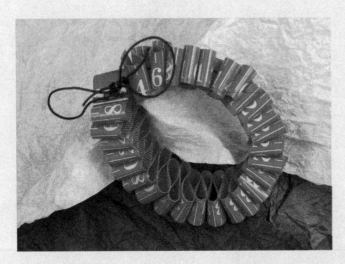

SUPPLIES

one needle with eye that is large enough to get the elastic thread through
black elastic thread
one tape measure (color of your choice, although the red with red nail polish makes a lovely combo)

INSTRUCTIONS

Thread your needle with the black elastic thread and knot it at the end. Place needle at the ½-inch mark and sew through, then loop the tape measure to the left and put the needle through at the ½-inch mark (and through at the 2.5-, 3.5-, 4.5-inch marks). Then loop to the right, putting the needle through at the next ½-inch mark. Keep zigzagging back and forth so the bracelet looks much like a ruffled collar. The needle is going through in the middle of the bracelet, not at the ends. When you get to the end of the tape measure, tie a knot and cut the elastic. Tie the ends together. The bracelet slips on and off, given its elasticity.

Our Lady of Chocolate Dreams

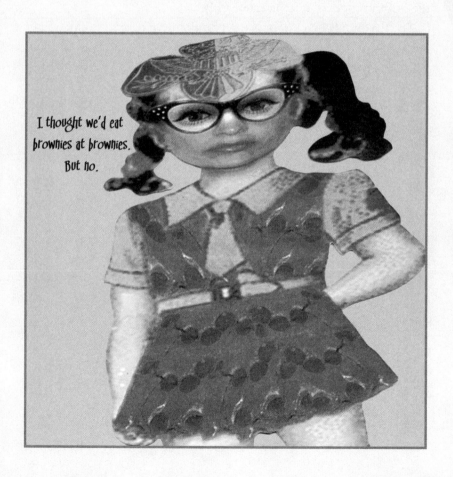

I thought we'd eat brownies at brownies. But no.

"Nothing chocolate . . . nothing gained."
~Anonymous

fa T oid
The melting point of
cocoa butter is just
below the human body's
average temperature—
which is why it actually
melts in your mouth.

MOTIVATIONAL MUSING
Hey, Kids

Hold on to your chocolate bar. Dark chocolate that is—and listen up. Dark chocolate (that's chocolate minus the milk) is now proclaimed the healthy chocolate, to be eaten daily.

The flavonoids in a 1.6 ounce serving of dark chocolate a day for a two-week period can help make your blood less sticky. Dark chocolate keeps your arteries supple. It helps heal injuries inside the blood vessels. It therefore reduces the risk of heart attack.

A word to the wise: If you are happily including 1.6 ounces of dark chocolate a day in your food plan, remember that it has calories, and too many calories consumed results in weight gain. Be sure to keep track of what you are eating and stay within your calorie/point/gram allotments.

Tasty Tidbit one ounce of dark chocolate

Calories: 170	Fat grams: 14
Protein grams: 4	Saturated-fat grams: 0
Carbohydrate grams: 9	Cholesterol milligrams: 0
Sodium milligrams: 0	Percent fat calories: 77
Fiber grams: 0	

WEIGHTY CONFESSION

Forgive Me for I Have Sinned

I believe in my heart of hearts that it is a sin to throw away chocolate. So, I searched high and low for some deserving person to give the stash of chocolate bars that I uncovered in the back of the fridge. Alas, no one deserving presented themselves, so I ate them—all!

All Is Forgiven.
Move On.

Dear Our Lady of Weight Loss,

I have been enjoying your newsletter for a few months. Because of your inspiration and a wandering rodent, I put all of my dark chocolate into a tin, which I promptly forgot about. At the end of last week, I was to go on a clear liquid diet prior to a medical test. The day before, I was searching for one good thing to eat before the fast began—my last hurrah—when I came across the tin. I slowly opened it. I felt like I was opening Pandora's box! I ate two pieces of chocolate. But you know what?! It didn't taste good! Wahoo! I am a reformed, recovering chocoholic. Thank you for all of your inspiration! Wow. I never thought I would say that any chocolate didn't taste good. You are too cool! ~Judy P

Dear Judy P,

Oh, my! Yuk—a rodent. I'm horrified. Killed my appetite for sure. Thank you!!!! 'Tis you who are cool. ~Our Lady of Weight Loss

Pious Project
BOX OF CHOCOLATE DREAMS

SWEET CHILDHOOD DREAMS

When I was a kid, my dad owned a pharmacy, and it was stocked with all kinds of candies—from Mars bars to Whitman's sampler boxes. The store was up the block from the elementary school that I attended. So, I would often leave school and head to the candy counter. Can you imagine? I could take whatever I wanted—for free!

There are so many sweet memories connected to Mars bars and Butterfingers. On special occasions I was allowed to treat myself to a small Whitman's sampler box. I loved the map. I would read it over and over again, deciding which candy to eat first, and which to offer to friends (cream centers weren't my favorites).

Recently, my friend Tina gave me an empty Whitman's box. The map is now written in three languages: English, French, and Spanish.

Solid Chocolate Messenger Boy

Le messager en chocolat solide

Nino mensajero de chocolate de leche macio

This box of candy is dedicated to the delicious memory of my sweet daddy.

SUPPLIES

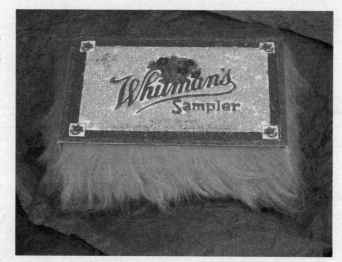

- one *empty* box of Whitman Samplers (Empty as in your friend donated a box to your Pious Project efforts, not as in you ate it!)
- glitter glue
- craft cement glue
- seed beads
- faux fur
- double-sided tape
- big round balls or beads (for the feet)

INSTRUCTIONS

Paint the words "Whitman's Sampler" with the glitter glue (bright color of your choice), and the trim around the outside of the top of the box. When dry, give it another coat. Squeeze the cement glue, an inch or so at a time, on the area on the top of the box where there are no words. Generously place seed beads on top of cement glue.

Measure box and cut fur to fit the sides.

Take double-sided tape and run along the top of the sides of the box. Place faux fur on it.

To make feet, glue large beads to the bottom four corners of the box. I had a stash of old-school electric typewriter balls. I'd been saving them for years, and thought this box was "old-school" worthy!

I use the inside of the box to store my favorite earrings. The trays are perfect for them.

Kick No. 12

Our Lady Puts One Foot in Front of the Other

"The sedentary life is the very sin against the Holy Spirit. Only thoughts reached by walking have value."

~Friedrich Nietzche

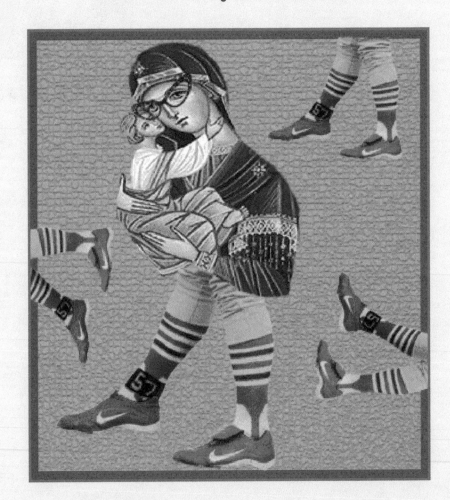

The Benefits of Walking

faToid

Walking an extra twenty
minutes each day will
burn off seven pounds
of body fat per year.

From stress reduction to less incidence of cancer, heart disease, stroke, and diabetes, the benefits of walking are amazing! Some even say walking relieves constipation and helps cure impotence.

Walking stimulates the brain to release endorphins and increases the production of the neurotransmitter serotonin, the body's natural mood elevator. Literally, walking makes us happy.

Richard Carmona, U.S. Surgeon General, advises, "Walking is the biggest bang for our buck. Thirty minutes a day of walking will prevent many cases of diabetes, hypertension, and other chronic diseases. Walking is the simplest, easiest way [to exercise] for most people."

And Secretary of Health and Human Services Tommy Thompson logs in ten thousand steps a day on his pedometer.

Even Thomas Jefferson, author of the Declaration of Independence and third president of the United States, believed that "of all exercises, walking is the best."

It seems to be our patriotic duty is to walk!

Here are a few ideas from Our Lady of Weight Loss on how to increase your daily steps:

- Get off the bus or subway one stop earlier than usual.
- Park your car at the far end of the mall.
- Dust and/or vacuum your home during commercials (especially during the food commercials).

- Take the stairs instead of the elevator.
- Get up and go visit coworkers. Resist the urge to use the intercom or e-mail.
- Pick up lunch instead of ordering out.
- Walk your neighbor's dog! (He'll like you for it!)
- Wear a pedometer! It will keep you honest, and you can compete against yourself daily!

Tasty Tidbit **Walking tip: Do your thighs rub together as you walk, creating a bit of chafing irritation? Don't sweat it. You're not alone. Try sprinkling a bit of powder on those prime meat spots and wear loose, comfortable clothing!**

WEIGHTY CONFESSION
Forgive Me for I Have Sinned

I spend a good deal of time on the sofa, shouting for my kids to bring me this and that, directing all who are nearby, never leaving my seat if not absolutely necessary. And yet, I feel that life is unfair and unjust. However did my tush get so big?

All Is Forgiven.
Move On.

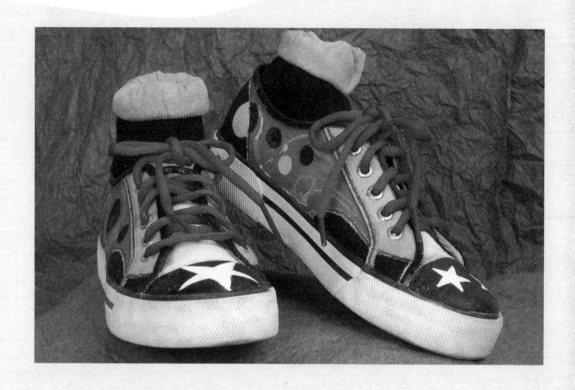

Pious Project
OUR LADY FLYERS

Are you having one of those days where you just can't get going? Your mind is saying, "Walk, walk, walk." But your body is saying, "Sleep, sleep, sleep." You need a boost!

Paint yourself a pair of snappy, colorful, and magical Our Lady Flyers. Get jazzed. Get moving!

SUPPLIES

one pair of old sneakers

double-sided craft tape in the shape of round circles and stars

size 1 and size 2 paintbrushes

fabric paint: yellow, orange, purple, black

small ice tray or painter's tray

red shoe laces

glass of water to clean brushes

paper towels (always a good idea to have handy in case of spills)

INSTRUCTIONS

Clean off sneakers. You don't want round dust balls mixed in with wet paint (trust me).

Place different-size double-sided tape circles and stars randomly on your sneakers. They act as a "resist," as the parts covered resist the paint. My sneakers already had a great pattern, so I followed the stitching and grids. Once again, it's like coloring, but this time you're using fabric paint.

Paint the stitches one color. And then paint the different sections of the sneakers different colors.

Paint around the circles and stars. If they are lying securely on the fabric, they should prevent the paint from getting underneath.

Once dry, you can either remove the top protective layer of the double-sided tape and sprinkle beads or sparkles onto it (although the beads et al. are not rainproof). Or, as I did, remove the tape entirely and paint the circles and stars contrasting colors with the fabric paint.

Lace up and let them take you on a power walk!

Kick No. 13

Our Lady of the Skinfully Beautiful

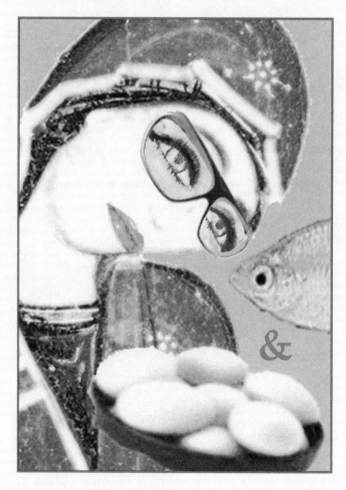

"I'm tired of all this nonsense about beauty being only skin-deep. That's deep enough. What do you want—an adorable pancreas?"

~Jean Kerr

"The brain and skin are deeply connected from the earliest moments of life. Touch is one of the first senses to develop. Even in the womb, a baby feels its way to bring hand to mouth."

~*National Geographic*

MOTIVATIONAL MUSING
Beauty's Only Skin Deep, Ya, Ya, Ya

Like the heart, stomach, and brain, your skin is an organ. In fact, it's the largest organ in your body, and it grows from the inside out. Its primary purpose is to protect what's inside.

There are many nutrients, including protein, vitamins, minerals, healthy fats, and water that are needed to condition, repair, and regenerate your skin.

Water, sometimes called the forgotten nutrient, rids your body of toxins and keeps skin moist. Be sure to drink approximately half your body weight in ounces per day. (If you weigh 150 pounds that would mean that you need to drink approximately 9 glasses of water per day.)

For healthy and beautiful skin, here's the A, B, C skinny on the subject:

Vitamin A helps to even out skin tone and diminish fine lines, and may help to make your skin more elastic. Good sources are: egg yolks, milk and dairy products, fish oil.

Vitamin B controls oil secretion, decreases propensity toward blemishes, and helps to prevent scaly skin. Sources: Poultry, fish, whole grains, dried beans, bananas, meat, leafy green veggies, as well as dairy products.

Vitamin C helps heal scar tissue and cuts and bruises, and protects against UVA rays. Sources: citrus fruits, broccoli, cabbage, tomatoes, berries, melon, peppers, potatoes.

Vitamin D helps to moisturize and condition skin. Sources: egg yolks, salmon, herring, and fortified milk.

Vitamin E conditions and moisturizes skin, helps heal burns, inflammation, cuts, and irritation, and may minimize formation of scars. Sources: wheat germ, nuts, vegetable oil, green leafy vegetables, whole grains.

Essential fatty acids moisturize the skin while helping to maintain its barrier function. Sources: flaxseed oil, evening primrose oil, black currants, safflower oil, borage seed oil, linoleic acid.

Vitamin K reduces bruising, may help relieve dark circles under eyes, treats actinic purpura in aged skin, and may help fade broken capillaries. Sources: green leafy vegetables.

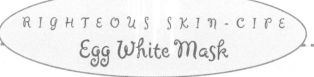

R I G H T E O U S   S K I N - C I P E
Egg White Mask

NOT FOR CONSUMPTION!!!

Ingredients

    one egg

Directions

    Break open the egg and separate the white from the yolk.

    Beat the white for one minute with whisk. Gently apply this whisked white wonder to your skin and let it harden. Wash it off with warm water. The egg white draws toxins from the skin's surface and tightens the pores as it cleans.

Dear Our Lady of Weight Loss,

Is it okay to use olive oil as a moisturizer straight from the bottle? As expensive as olive oil can be, it's still a lot less than those fancy crèmes. What do you think?
~Olive Oyl, Lover of Popeye

Dear Olive Oyl,

I've heard that olive oil is good for the skin. You might want to add a couple of drops of lavender essential oil to it. It's also great for the skin and the aroma is calming. Ahhh. And remember that eating foods with the proper nutrients is key!
~Our Lady of Weight Loss

Our Lady of Lustrous Locks

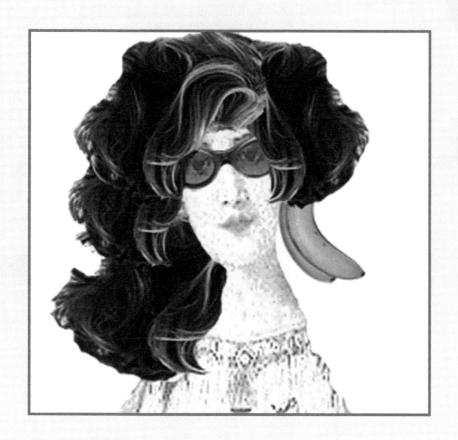

"Does she . . .
or doesn't she?"
~Clairol hair color
advertisement

MOTIVATIONAL MUSING
Whatta Hedda Hair

"Hair . . . shining, gleaming, streaming, flaxen, waxen . . ."
Your hairstyle creates an immediate and long-lasting impression.

To make the most of your hair, you need to understand it.

What Is Hair?

Hair is more or less a waste product that is eliminated from under the skin. It is made up of a protein called keratin (which is also responsible for the elasticity of fingernails).

Only a healthy head produces healthy hair.

What to Do?

The **first step** is to make sure you're eating enough foods that are heavy in the B vitamins, as well as a dash of A, C, and the omegas!

Here is a list of some hair-healthy foods that you might want to incorporate into your menu.

For **normal growth,** incorporate foods with B vitamins into your day. These include bananas, whole grains, fish, spinach, orange juice. The Bs help to form red blood cells, which carry oxygen to the hair!

To maintain a **healthy scalp and healthy hair** be sure to include milk and eggs, rich in Vitamin A, in your diet.

To **avoid hair breakage** try one cup of broccoli and/or a cup of orange juice from freshly squeezed oranges (no sugar added) on a regular basis, both good sources of vitamin C.

Want **to rid yourself of dandruff?** Try foods heavy in zinc, such as oysters, poultry, beans, and fortified cereals.

For **hair pigmentation** (strong color) include the fatty fishes (salmon and sardines), chicken, turkey, eggs, and soy foods in your plan.

The **second step** is to get yourself a good stylist!

Tasty Tidbit Here are some tips on how to have sexy hair (not that I adhere to any of them).

Simplicity rules. Try an uncomplicated clean cut with simple lines.

Don't hide behind your hair. It's okay to show your face. Really. You're okay.

You're never going to look like Madonna. Even if your stylist can cut your hair just like your favorite celeb, you won't look like her.

Get a makeup makeover. If you're wearing blue eye shadow, the best, sexiest hair cut in the world ain't gonna help you.

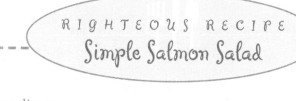

RIGHTEOUS RECIPE
Simple Salmon Salad

Ingredients

1 lb. salmon fillet, poached and cooled to room temperature

2 celery stalks, finely chopped

Nutrition Facts		
Serving Size (182g)		
Servings Per Container 4		
Amount Per Serving		
Calories 220	Calories from Fat 90	
		% Daily Value*
Total Fat 10g		**15%**
Saturated Fat 2g		**10%**
Trans Fat 0g		
Cholesterol 70mg		**23%**
Sodium 370mg		**15%**
Total Carbohydrate 6g		**2%**
Dietary Fiber 1g		**4%**
Sugars 2g		
Protein 26g		
Vitamin A 2%	•	Vitamin C 15%
Calcium 4%	•	Iron 8%

*Percent Daily Values are based on a 2,000 calorie diet. Your daily values may be higher or lower depending on your calorie needs:

		Calories	2,000	2,500
Total Fat	Less Than		65g	80g
Saturated Fat	Less Than		20g	25g
Cholesterol	Less Than		300mg	300 mg
Sodium	Less Than		2,400mg	2,400mg
Total Carbohydrate			300g	375g
Dietary Fiber			25g	30g

Calories per gram:
Fat 9 • Carbohydrate 4 • Protein 4

½ red onion, peeled, finely sliced

2 Tbs. of capers (strain out the pickling juice) (I love salty capers; you might want to put 1 Tbs. in and see how it tastes before adding the second.)

juice of 1 lemon (regular lemon, not Meyer lemon)

¼ cup reduced-fat mayo

2 Tbs. fresh dill, chopped

salt and freshly ground pepper

Directions

Combine all ingredients in bowl and serve, on light bread or on a bed of lettuce.

WEIGHTY CONFESSION
Forgive Me for I Have Sinned

I woke up in the middle of the night and headed straight to the kitchen. The refrigerator was just about bare, with the exception of a condiment or two. I was crazed and desperate. I ate two frozen hot dogs. No, I didn't bother to cook them. (Don't worry, I'm seeking counseling.)

All Is Forgiven.
Move On.

Kick No. 15

Our Lady of
Luminous Laughter

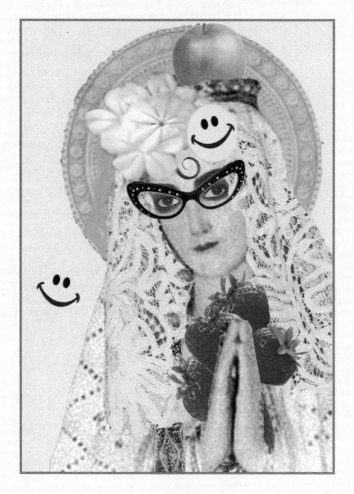

"If one is lucky,
a solitary fantasy
can totally
transform one
million realities."
~Maya Angelou

MOTIVATIONAL MUSING
Life Is a Laugh Fest

Laughing one hundred times is the equivalent to a ten-minute workout on the rowing machine or fifteen minutes on an exercise bike!

Laughter is made up of a series of short vowel-like sounds repeated every 210 milliseconds (one thousandth of a second). Laughter almost always occurs during a pause at the end of a phrase or at the end of a sentence. You either laugh in the "ho-ho-ho" style or the "ha-ha-ha" style, but your laughing mechanism won't mix the two.

Humor and laughter are two different things, and up to 80 percent of laughter is not in response to a joke! Women laugh 126 percent more often than men. (Are you surprised?) And there is evidence that laughter is medically beneficial.

While suffering from a collagen disease Norman Cousins checked into a hotel room and watched one funny movie after another. He laughed (despite his gender)! Mr. Cousins found that ten minutes of really big laughs gave him two pain-free hours of sleep. And he also found that laughter, in time, cured his disease. How amazing is that?

Laughter makes us feel good both physiologically and psychologically.

Laughter~
- ◆ **reduces** levels of certain stress hormones.
- ◆ **reduces** anxiety and tension.
- ◆ **boosts** the immune system by stimulating the thymus gland.

- may lead to hiccupping but will **dislodge** mucus plugs from the respiratory tract! (How attractive!)
- **gives** you a full body, aerobic workout (works the diaphragm and abdominal, respiratory, facial, and back muscles).
- **gets** those positive endorphins pumping! Laughter invokes feelings of happiness and joy!
- **promotes** creative thoughts.
- **simulates** both sides of the brain.
- **creates bonding** with your fellow humans. Robert Provine, a neuroscientist at the University of Maryland, has studied laughter for more than a decade. Provine found that we laugh thirty times more often in social situations than when hanging solo. Nothing is better than a shared laugh!

Laughter is contagious. Spread it far and wide.

SACRED ASSIGNMENT
Laughter Is Contagious

Ready for a good laugh? Find a mirror and look into it. Your face is a reflection of your mind. What do you see? Relax into the inner you.

Smile at yourself. Be sure to smile with both your eyes and your mouth.

Close your eyes, breathe deep (in and out, in and out), relax your shoulders, smile gently, and feel your brain. Did you know that there's a direct connection from your heart to your brain? When your brain relaxes and rejoices, your heart dances.

Now—frown. As soon as you twist your face, your heart/brain connection gets blocked—your brain feels tense. As we know, smiling and laughing affect your brain in a positive way, so this makes sense.

Repeat this exercise a number of times; first smiling, then frowning. This stimulates your brain.

Now laugh as hard as you can. Shake your every part of your body. Focus on your face, then your chest, your belly, your knees, and finally your toes, laughing all the while.

A good laugh opens your energy center.

Are you brimming over with energy and joy?

Dear Our Lady of Weight Loss,

I have always been heavy. I started gaining weight in the womb—well, I guess we all did—but mine was an extreme case. I weighed in at over eleven pounds at birth, and it's been uphill (or downhill) since then. I can't imagine that I could ever be thin. Would you be kind enough to imagine it for me? ~Forever Fat

Dear Fat No More *(formerly known as Forever Fat),*

I can see your inner-thinner core without difficulty. So yes, I am more than happy to help you visualize yourself as a thin person. Our first step is to give you a new name. Henceforth, you shall be known as Fat No More. I will add you to my Daily Visualization List. (Yes, it's kind of like a daily prayer list.) Seeing oneself as thin takes practice and diligence. It's like building a muscle. It's important you participate as well. Our Lady helps those who help themselves. So, let's be sure to dedicate a few minutes every day to visualize the best for ourselves and for our loved ones. We can exercise our visualization muscles together.

~Our Lady of Weight Loss

Pious Project
JEWEL BOX

Boxes are alluring. What do they hold? A secret love note? The family pound cake recipe? Your diamond tiara? When I ate the last (Laughing Cow) low-fat triangle cheese and was left with an empty round box, I realized I had struck weight-loss D.I.Y. craft project *gold!*

I turned the box into a sacrosanct holder of my jewels. (My rings—some are from the supermarket's bubble gum machine that I had the cheap thrill of purchasing for only twenty-five cents, but nevertheless priceless.)

You can keep your sacred jewels or beatific buttons (Pious Project, page 125) in your round creation.

SUPPLIES

glitter tape

1 round box (I used Laughing Cow's light cheese box)

sponge brush

hot pink tempera paint

light green glitter glue

pink seed beads

dry green split peas

paintbrush, size 1 is fine

craft cement glue

plastic flower

four gorgeous beads that the box can sit on (aka feet)

INSTRUCTIONS

The graphics from the original box are colorful and appealing, so I left the bottom half as is. You can too, or paint over—it's all art! (Oh, what a great expression.)

Run the self-adhering glitter tape around the side of the box top.

Using your sponge brush, wistfully brush the hot pink paint around the top outer edge. A light touch, please—nothing heavy handed.

Next, we're going to fill in the top of the box.

Squeeze a layer of light green glitter glue straight from the bottle.

Sprinkle a mixture of pink seed beads and dry green peas over it. (Since the glitter glue is a glue with glitter, it will hold the seed beads and green peas.)

Using craft cement, glue the plastic flower smack in the middle of the top.

When the top is dry, it's time to move on to the feet.

Dab a spot of cement glue on the top of each bead and place the box on top of them, so that they are of equal distance from each other and serve as legs.

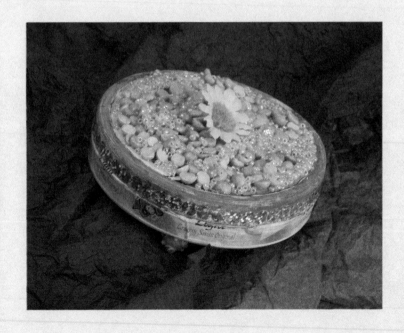

Prickly Prayer

Dear Our Lady of Weight Loss,
Now I lay me down to sleep.
I pray Our Lady my fat to keep.
But should I dine before I wake,
I pray Our Lady to set me straight!

Amen.

Kick No. 16

Our Lady of the Sacred Snooze

"Sleep is the golden chain that ties health and our bodies together."
~Thomas Dekker

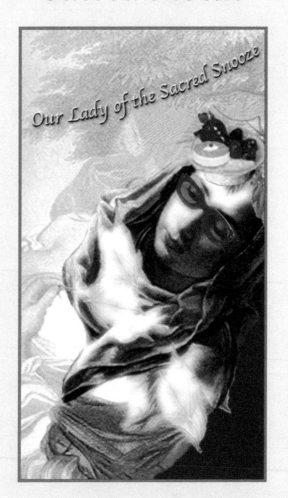

Our Lady of the Sacred Snooze

104

Chronic Sleep Deprivation Can Make You *Fat*!

Snooze and Lose

fa**T**oid

If you fall asleep in anything less than five minutes at night, it means you're sleep deprived. Ideally, it should take you between ten and fifteen minutes. You are tired enough to sleep deeply, but not so exhausted you feel sleepy by day.

Sleep plays a crucial part in weight loss. The less sleeping hours you log in, the more likely you are to expand—that's your waist and your thighs, not your horizons!

Lack of sleep causes our body to produce lower levels of an appetite-regulating hormone (leptin), and higher levels of a hormone produced by the stomach that sends out hunger signals to the brain (ghrelin). These hormones regulate our metabolism and let us know when we are full.

In other words, lack of sleep causes hormonal changes that tell you to eat. These hormonal changes may also signal the body to slow its metabolism and to hold on to the fats. (What a wacky system!) Bottom line: Make sure you get sufficient sleep.

Lack of sleep also increases your risk for heart attack and lessens the release of serotonin, the pleasure hormone from your brain. To make yourself feel better, you are likely to reach for foods with high levels of sugar.

Sleep recharges the entire system, including your eyes. Sleep allows your retinal membranes to recharge after a hard day of seeing. Be sure to take ten breaks from the computer every two hours!

How Much Sleep Should You Get?

Men should get a minimum of seven to eight hours of sleep every night, and women, six to seven hours.

Having Trouble Sleeping?

- Limit your caffeine intake (coffee, tea, and chocolate!).
- Limit alcohol and do *not* drink right before bedtime. It may make you sleepy; however, alcohol disrupts REM sleep.
- Create a relaxing bedtime ritual: light candles and incense, meditate, think healthy thoughts.
- Take a hot bath, breathe deep, listen to restful music.
- Eliminate nighttime worry. Shelve the negative thoughts for the morning!
- Take your siesta early in the day, not too close to nighttime.
- Add the following fruits to your food plan: papaya, banana, strawberries, sweet cherries, oranges, mangoes, pineapple.

Tasty Tidbit **Those who sleep less than four hours a night are 73 percent more likely to be obese than those who sleep seven to nine hours.**

Dear Our Lady of Weight Loss,

I'm exhausted. Exhausted from dieting, from life, from lack of sleep. All I want to do is eat. Help! ~*Sleepless-in-Somnia*

Dear Sleepless-In-Somnia,

Sounds like you need a good night's sleep, a vacation, and some fruits and vegetables. Oh, and water and exercise, too. Lack of sleep, good food, and water can make us feel depressed, hopeless, and hungry. My advice: Take a nice long walk. Clear your head. Renew your commitment to yourself. ~Our Lady of Weight Loss

Tasty Tidbit **It's true! If you drink a glass of warm milk fifteen minutes before bedtime, those jangled nerves will smooth right out. Ahhhh.**

RIGHTEOUS RECIPE
Banana Strawberry Sleep-Time Custard

This recipe is for those of us whose sweet tooth takes up their entire mouth. It's very sweet and a good substitute for custard, cake, or candy. It's not exactly custard, but hey—I like it.

Ingredients

nonstick spray

6 egg whites, beaten

½ cup of sugar blend (it's ½ sugar, ½ artificial sweetener)

1 generous tsp. vanilla extract

1 12-oz. can fat-free skim evaporated milk

Nutrition Facts

Serving Size (433g)
Servings Per Container 6

Amount Per Serving

Calories 270   Calories from Fat 10

	% Daily Value*
Total Fat 1g	2%
Saturated Fat 0g	0%
Trans Fat 0g	
Cholesterol 5mg	2%
Sodium 480mg	20%
Total Carbohydrate 34g	11%
Dietary Fiber 3g	12%
Sugars 26g	
Protein 32g	

Vitamin A 6%	•	Vitamin C 80%
Calcium 20%	•	Iron 4%

*Percent Daily Values are based on a 2,000 calorie diet. Your daily values may be higher or lower depending on your calorie needs:

	Calories	2,000	2,500
Total Fat	Less Than	65g	80g
Saturated Fat	Less Than	20g	25g
Cholesterol	Less Than	300mg	300 mg
Sodium	Less Than	2,400mg	2,400mg
Total Carbohydrate		300g	375g
Dietary Fiber		25g	30g

Calories per gram:
Fat 9 • Carbohydrate 4 • Protein 4

---

1 tsp. cream of tartar

2 bananas

1 16-oz. container fresh strawberries

Directions

Preheat oven to 325°.

Spray 8" baking pan with nonstick spray.

In a large bowl, whisk egg whites, add sugar blend, vanilla, evaporated milk, and cream of tartar.

Pour mixture into pan and bake at 325° for 40 minutes—or until custard is a light brown. Remove from oven.

Let cool.

Slice bananas and strawberries and place on top, in a pretty pattern. "It's all art!"

Pious Project
GOAL PIN

When you reach your weight-loss goal, celebrate by giving yourself a major rock. I did!

SUPPLIES

major diamonds (available at craft store)

cement glue

one tin heart shape (available at craft stores)

seed beads (gold)

pin back

INSTRUCTIONS

Strategically glue your diamonds onto the tin heart shape by putting a dab of cement glue on their flat side.

Squeeze a light layer of cement glue on the rest of the pin and generously sprinkle with seed beads.

When dry, flip over, and using cement, glue the pin back in place (a quarter of the way down, so it lies on your blouse gracefully).

Walla! You've given yourself a major rock of self-appreciation.

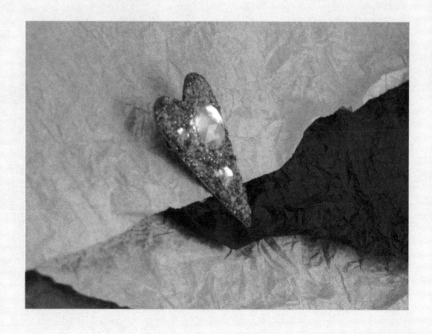

Our Lady Says Grace

"Grace is to the
body what good
manners are to
the mind."

~ François de La
Rochefoucauld

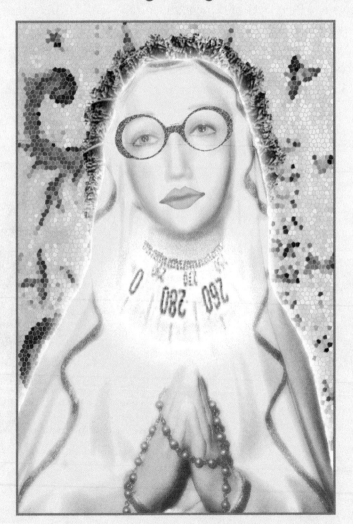

MOTIVATIONAL MUSING
Minding Grace

faToid

"Amazing Grace" is one
of the most popular
hymns in the English
language.

We have a built-in system that tells our brain when we've had enough to eat. It's call satiety. However, we're very skilled at overriding it! How do we do this? We eat really, really fast.

It takes twenty minutes before our brain catches up to our stomach and realizes that it's full. So, when we eat too fast, our brain doesn't realize that we've downed 800 calories in three minutes. It thinks we're still hungry, so we keep on eating. I don't know about you, but I can do a whole lot of damage in twenty minutes.

Eating fast puts us at risk for acid reflux, choking, and weight gain!

What to do? Slow down and eat with mindfulness. You know, consciousness. That means no reading or watching television while eating, or talking on the phone. Eating with mindfulness can help us to taste and enjoy our meal, while at the same time the stress from our day dissipates into the universe.

One of my preferred ways to slow things down before they even get started is to say grace. Saying grace is a universal form of spiritual nourishment; a shared type of spoken prayer. And grace sets the tone of the meal and reminds me of my intention: to slow my pace, to appreciate the bounty of the food on my table, to remember that life is not a race, but rather a gift.

The Our Lady of Weight Loss's
One-Minute Manual to Grace

Authenticity counts. There's no right or wrong way to say grace, as long as it comes from your heart.

The logistics. Should I sit or stand? Should I bow my head or look up? Should we all hold hands or not? Again, there's no right or wrong. Do whatever feels the most comfortable.

Who will say grace? If you're alone that's an easy one! But if not, you might want to ask the eldest, or the youngest, or if clergy is present (I grew up down the block from a convent and Our Lady of Snow, so clergy was an easy thing to come by), ask him or her to do the honors.

What to say? You might want to recite a standard prayer from the religion of your choice or words that feel appropriate for the occasion. Consider who is at the table. If there are a lot of fidgety children at the table, keep it short!

Pious Project
GRACE'S PLACE (CARDS)

SUPPLIES
place card for each person at the table
heavy colored paper stock (4" x 6")

heavyweight white paper (3.75" x 5.75")
scissors with wiggly cut
pretty calligraphy pens or paint pens
prayer to copy
glitter, stars, stamp pads, whatever you like

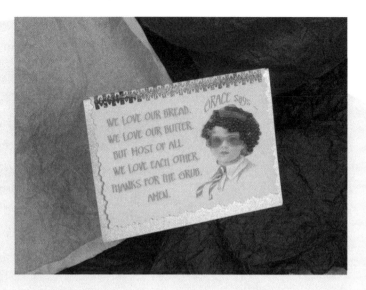

HERE ARE SOME SAMPLE PRAYERS OF GRACE

Christian prayer. "Be present at our table, Lord; be here, and everywhere adored; thy mercies bless and grant that we may feast in fellowship with thee. Amen."

Jewish prayer. "Blessed art thou O Lord my G-d, king of the universe, who brings forth the bread from the earth."

Sufi prayer. "O Thou, the Sustainer of our bodies, hearts, and souls, bless all that we receive in thankfulness."

Preschool prayer. "We love our bread. We love our butter. But most of all, we love each other, Thanks for the grub. Amen"

INSTRUCTIONS

You can either use preexisting place cards that you've purchased from your favorite stationery store, or make your own.

First, fold your heavy stock 4" x 6" paper in the middle, forming a tent.

Print out (or hand write) your favorite prayer (image on it optional) on the bottom half of your white (or light) stock paper that measures 3.75" x 5.75" (it's slightly smaller than your tent). You can cut a wiggly border with your special scissors.

Fold and place on tent card, so that the prayer is in the front.

Glitter tape makes a nice trim across the top and also holds it in place.

WEIGHTY CONFESSION

Forgive Me for I Have Sinned

I've been trying to say grace for over three weeks now, but as soon as I see the food, my mind, body, and soul go straight to it, and I forget. I'll keep trying.

All Is Forgiven.

Move On.

Dear Our Lady of Weight Loss,

Please help. My husband and I separated last summer, and I've put on some weight. I have suffered through a few surgeries, (back, neck, and knees)—one two days before he left. What can I do to get my heart, head, and body to go forward with renewed strength, comfort, and flexibility? I am doing well to walk. I am an art teacher for 450 wonderfully loving K–6 artists. ~Ready to Paint a New, Free Me

Dear Ready to Paint,

I'm so sorry that you've been through such a rough time. My advice would be to focus your loving, kind energy on those 450 wonderful K–6 grade kids and yourself! Paint your woes away. Walk a little farther every day. Stretch your arms into the vast, blue skies and smile. Onward and upward. We're rootin' for you every step of the way! ~Our Lady of Weight Loss

PS: We won't speak of the man.

Prickly Prayer

Dear Our Lady of the Deep Cleansing Breath,

May I inhale thin
and exhale fat.
Thin in; fat out.
Thin in; fat out.
Fat out—out—out.

Amen.

Kick No. 18

Our Lady of the Deep Cleansing Breath

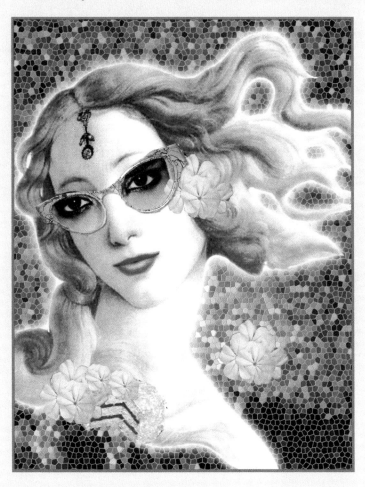

"Breathe-in
experience,
breathe-out
poetry."
~"Poem Out of
Childhood,"
Muriel Rukeyser

MOTIVATIONAL MUSING
Breathe Deep

Our weight depends on a complicated blend of variables, from how much we move (exercise), to what we eat, how much we eat, how we feel about ourselves, to hereditary factors. Our weight is even linked to how we breathe. We should breathe in six quarts of air per minute.

Breathing can

- affect our metabolism;
- affect the quantity of food we ingest;
- make us feel better mentally, physically, and emotionally;
- calm us;
- release endorphins, which help us to feel happy;
- enhance our appearance;
- make us feel instantly stronger and thinner;
- revitalize and energize every cell in our bodies;
- increase our energy level.

Deep breathing can aid our weight-loss effort. Healthy breathing helps us maintain the right balance of oxygen and carbon dioxide in our cells, which has a favorable impact on our metabolism.

Dr. Jon Kabat-Zinn, an author, says, "Every breath, actually, is a release not only of air, but all the pent-up energy in the body. Every in-breath can be restoration or revitalization, and every out-breath a letting-go of anxiety or anger or tension or irritability."

Instead of stuffing down your feelings with food, breathe. It's natural. It's calorie-free. And it's easy.

SACRED ASSIGNMENT

Deep Breath

1. Begin by either lying flat on your back, standing up straight and tall, or sitting up straight in a chair. Whatever works for you. Personally, I think it's always best to be horizontal.
2. Place your hands on your stomach. (Try not to get caught up in feeling just how big or soft it is. We're here to breathe, not judge or torment.)
3. Breathe the way you normally do. Is your hand rising with your breath or is your chest rising?
4. To breathe properly, your stomach area must rise as your diaphragm expands.
5. Begin by slowly breathing in through your nose on the count of five while gently pushing your hand up with your stomach.
6. Hold the breath for a count of five.
7. Slowly exhale through your mouth for a count of five while gently pushing down on your stomach.
8. Repeat this process for five minutes. If five minutes is too much for you to start, start with one minute.

9. Increase the length of time each time you do this breathing exercise. Ultimately, it would be great if you could breathe for five minutes twice a day.

10. The more you practice mindful breathing, the more likely you are to do it naturally throughout the day.

WEIGHTY CONFESSION

Forgive Me for I Have Sinned

I fear that I have sunk down to a new all-time weigh-in low. I was going to my group meeting—wherein we weigh in—and to ensure the lowest possible numbers, I painstakingly assembled the appropriate weigh-in outfit. I rolled up all my shorts, tops, bras, and panties, and one by one weighed them on my food scale. Just so you know, thong underwear weighs an entire 1 ounce less than full bikinis.

All Is Forgiven.
Move On.

Pious Project
BUBBLE PURSE

Want to add that special accessory to your already fabulous outfit? Whip up a bubble purse!

SUPPLIES

mesh bag that holds oranges (the next time you go to the supermarket, keep an eye peeled for oranges or potatoes that are packaged in mesh bags. Buy them!)

bubble wrap (about a yard)

cement glue

dried peas or beans (also from the supermarket)

paper flowers on wire stems; two dozen should be more than enough (Crafts stores have them, or fancy paper stores.)

orange taffeta (2½ yds.)

INSTRUCTIONS

Be careful when you open the bag. You'll want to keep the tag attached, as it will serve as the bottom of your bag.

Remove oranges or potatoes!

Tuck the mesh (from the open side of the bag) inside the bag, keeping the tag on the bottom.

The size of your bag will depend on the size of your mesh.

Fold the mesh inward until you get the bag size you like.

Measure its height and circumference (my bag was 6" high and 7" wide and 4" deep) and cut the bubble wrap in one long piece accordingly for the sides. Place it inside the mesh, forming the inner lining.

Measure the bottom of the bag. (Mine was 7" x 4") Cut two 7" x 4"

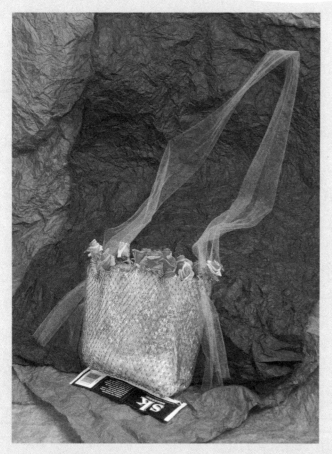

pieces of bubble wrap. You are going to make a "bean sandwich." On one of the pieces of bubble wrap squeeze some cement glue and sprinkle generously with beans; add a little cement to the top and put the top piece of bubble wrap on it. Then place it on the bottom of the bag. The weight of the beans helps to give the bag its shape. Let it dry.

Next take the wire stem of a flower and pierce it through the mesh and bubble wrap and twist it until the flower is sitting right on the rim. Distribute the flowers evenly around the top rim of the bag.

Now we are going to make the handle. Punch a hole with any sharp object on the side of your bag, about ½" down. Repeat on the opposite side. Pull the taffeta through on one side. Knot it there, then on the other side, forming a strap. My piece of taffeta is about 2½ yards long. Tie a knot on each side, holding it in place.

Ready? Put your lipstick, cell phone, keys, and money in your purse—and go!

Kick No. 19

Our Lady Stands by Her Man

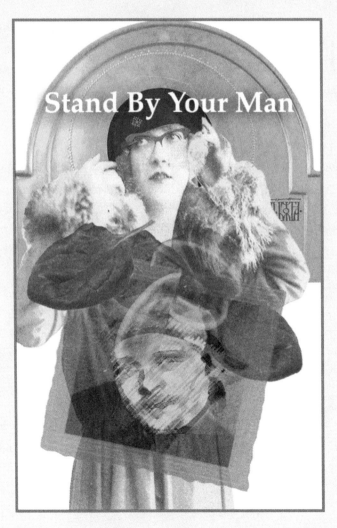

Stand By Your Man

" 'Cause after all,
he's just a man."
~"Stand by
Your Man,"
Tammy Wynette

faToid

Men who average
twenty-one orgasms a
month reduce their risk
of prostate cancer by
33 percent versus those
who average four to
seven orgasms
per month.

MOTIVATIONAL MUSING
Stand by Your Man

Want to keep your man healthy and happy? Feed him lots of foods containing lypocene and other carotenoids, including beta-carotene and lutein. These are the plant pigments that give the bright color to fruits and vegetables. The brighter and more colorful the diet, the healthier.

Foods that are good for your man include watermelon, tomatoes, pumpkin, citrus fruits, and spinach.

If your man eats just one 3 or 4 ounce serving of watermelon or pink grapefruit a day, he can reduce his risk of developing prostate cancer by 82 percent. Astounding! (Source: *International Journal of Cancer*)

A study by the USDA showed that watermelons have 40 percent more lypocene than tomatoes and do not need cooking to make their lypocene as readily available to the body. Conversely, tomatoes, when cooked or made into juice (something to do with the processing), yield more usable lypocene than watermelon. So crack open those watermelons, and get the tomato sauce bubbling!

Ply your man with brightly colored fruit, a nice red wine, and let's not forget the sex. Make him your superman!

Tasty Tidbit **One 4-ounce glass of antioxidant-rich red wine per week can reduce risk of prostate cancer by 50 percent! Source: Fred Hutchinson Cancer Research Center, Seattle, Washington**

Dear Our Lady of Weight Loss,

I sometimes think I am beyond all help. I need to lose one hundred pounds, and I have lost fifty to sixty pounds about ten times before. Imagine what that has done to my heart!! I have been this heavy since the birth of my daughter thirteen years ago. I know exactly what to do. I just can't seem to do it. I pray, I scream, I swear at myself. I have overcome life-threatening illnesses with a determination to get well, yet I can't stop eating. Any advice from anyone is very welcome. Thank you all.
~Can't Stop

Dear Can't Stop,

You can stop eating! There is always hope. You've just got to commit to the process, and no matter how long it takes, stick with it. Don't think of the other times as failures. Learn from them. Every time you have a negative thought, replace it with a positive thought. Every time you tell yourself that you can't do it, say, Yes, I can! Make healthy choices a lifestyle. Don't think of it as dieting. Diets don't work. But lifestyle changes do. Throw out all the crap you've probably got in your kitchen, and start anew. Not tomorrow. Right now! This time is your time!
~Our Lady of Weight Loss

Pious Project
BEATIFIC BUTTONS

In need of instant art gratification? What could be better than a bounty of beatific buttons?

Fast and easy, and they satiate—a beatific button is beautiful!

You can sew them on clothes, pocketbooks, embellish just about anything with them, or keep them in a bowl and look at them.

button-making kit (sewing shops have them)

images that please you—maybe a photo of your man?

heat-transfer paper (a more artistic way of saying T-shirt transfer paper or iron transfer paper)

½ yard of satin, silk, or cotton

INSTRUCTIONS

Read the instructions on the back of the button kit. The size of the buttons will determine the size of your images.

Pick out images that you'd like to put on your buttons. Choose images—from magazines, family photos, your man, or your own art—that you'd like to see on your buttons. You can print the images on your own computer or take them to your local print shop, give them the transfer paper, and they'll print them on the paper for you.

In order to put images on your fabric, you'll need to follow the directions on your heat-transfer paper package.

Now, follow the instructions on the back of your button kit to pop the fabric into place.

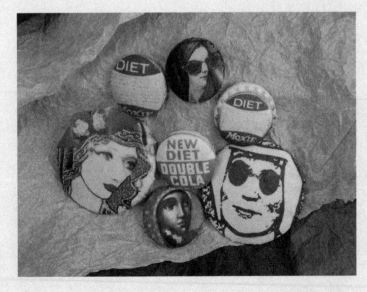

Our Lady's Evil Twin

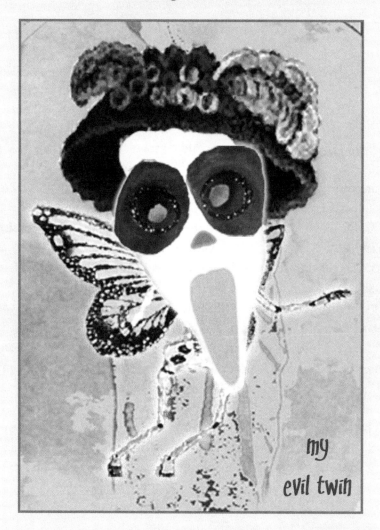

my
evil twin

"You were born together, and together you shall be forevermore ... but let there be spaces in your togetherness. And let the winds of the heavens dance between you."
~Kahlil Gibran

MOTIVATIONAL MUSING
The Inner Critic: aka My Evil Twin

We all have an evil twin that lives within, lurking in the background, waiting for an opportunity to rush to the forefront of our minds and lay the voice of chastisement on us.

My evil twin is quite convincing. She appears most often when I am entering new terrain. She is quite accomplished at mocking my desires to try new things. (Like permanently removing over fifty pounds, and letting the best of me shine through.) She's quick to say that I'm not smart enough, pretty enough, rich enough, young enough, talented enough, or even tall enough. I'm just not good enough!

And as far as weight loss goes, she has pointed out that I have a slow metabolism (she doesn't even know what a metabolism really is), an insatiable need for bad foods, and fat genes on both sides of the family. She is a master at activating all my insecurities and fears.

I spent decades believing her. With her words came feelings of defeat and shame. And then I would say to myself, "I'm never going to . . . make it, do it, have it, be it." My evil twin would then recede quite contently once again to the recesses of my mind, and rest until my next attempt at being, doing, having.

I tried to stand up to her. But honestly, she's so accomplished and has been my evil twin since conception. It just never worked. And then I realized that she was an enigma. She had no name, face, or personality. She was very one-dimensional. She was just the critic. I began to think that there must be something more to her—something that I could work with to help quiet her.

So I closed my eyes and demanded that she come forward. And you know what, she wasn't nearly as scary as I imagined! In fact, at closer examination I found that she had a quirky side as well, and I began to see her attempts to deep-six me as rather amusing.

Tasty Tidbit How to Quiet Your Evil Twin

If you listen closely to your inner critic, you'll find that she often sounds eerily like long ago said words of teachers, friends, siblings, or parents. Their advice may have been helpful twenty or more years ago, but it's no longer relevant.

Positive self-talk reigns supreme. Each time your inner critic attempts to shoot you down, praise yourself. Say, "I am fabulous, now get lost."

When your inner critic gets in your way and stops you from moving forward, stop and pay attention. What is the underlying fear? Fear is just a feeling; it's not real. Push past it. Is it worth sacrificing your creativity or yourself?

Do not compare yourself to others. It's deadly. There is always going to be someone out there who is smarter, more talented, prettier. So what! Embrace your uniqueness. You are a masterpiece.

Form a mutual admiration society. Spend time with people who are supportive, who say nice things to you, who recognize your beauty — the true essence of who you are. (Yes, I am fabulous, and you are too!)

When your inner critic is loud and won't back off, just let her ramble on. If she's just a mass of criticism, smile sweetly, tell her that she may continue to speak if she likes, but not so loudly, please, and she may as well know there's no way you're giving up on you anytime soon! (La, la, la . . . I'm singing over you and cannot hear you!)

Dear Our Lady of Weight Loss,

I read your article in First magazine and you truly are an inspiration to me! I have lost fifty-five pounds, but unfortunately I've gained twenty back. It was easy losing it the first time, but this time is so rough. Your article reminded and reinforced to me that I need to keep busy doing other things . . . rather than eating! I think of food twenty-four hours a day, seven days a week! It's an obsession or something, I'm not sure why. My toughest time is at night, when I sit in front of the TV and watch Dr. Phil (I tape it during the day and watch it at night when I get home). I'm going to start sewing, scrapbooking, petting the cat, etc. . . . to keep my hands busy (and my mind occupied) instead of eating! I hope I can lose this twenty pounds again! Thanks for the inspiration. ~Miss No Name
P.S. You look wonderful—keep it up!

Dear Miss No Name,

Congratulate yourself—you only regained twenty, not the entire fifty-five, and you're taking control now. Consider it part of the process and learn from your missteps. Statistics show that those who weigh themselves regularly (before things get out of hand), keep track of their daily food intake (as in, write it down), and exercise have a much better chance at permanently removing weight. Pretty much no one does it the first time out. Great, great, great! That you're sewing, scrapbooking, and petting the cat. Keep those hands busy. I'm sure there's a correlation. Please send a jpg of your arts-and-crafts work, and/or a photo of you petting your cat for the "Our Lady's Community Garden Art Gallery." ~Our Lady of Weight Loss

Pious Project
SAY HELLO TO YOUR EVIL TWIN

Cut and paste, draw, paint, or write your way to freedom. Describe your evil twin. What does your evil twin look like, sound like? How does she walk and talk? Now make friends with her and have a good laugh—together!

As you can see, I took a photo of myself (after all, she is my twin) and did her up!

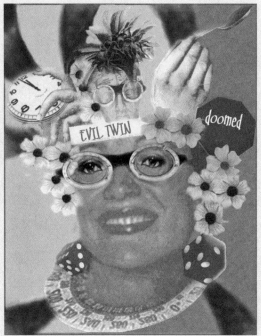

SUPPLIES

magazines
scissors
photocopy of photo of yourself
8" x 10" white paper
glue stick

INSTRUCTIONS

Go through a stack of magazines and rip out anything that you think would resonate with your evil twin. Both positive and negative images. Try not to think!

Place a photo of yourself on paper. Then go wild. Glue images and words under, over, and through your evil twin.

Now, look at your evil twin. What is she saying to you? Anything profound?

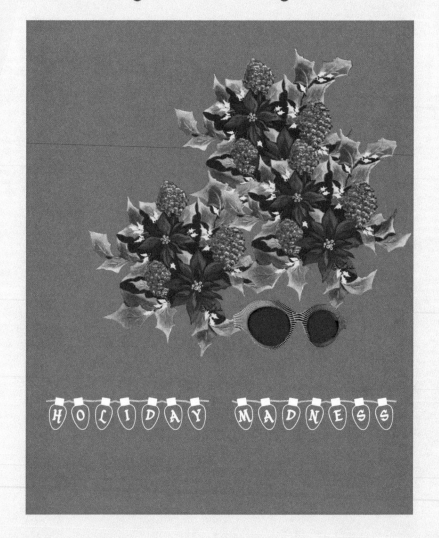

Kick No. 21

Our Lady of Holiday Madness

"Food to a large extent is what holds a society together and eating is closely linked to deep spiritual experiences."
~PeterGeorge FarbArmelagos

Ho, Ho—Hold On There!

faToid

The average weight gain during the holidays is just about one pound. However, we tend to hang on to that holiday pound—year after year after year.

It's easy to throw your hands up in the air and say, "It's okay. It's the holidays. I'll straighten up and eat right in January." But will you get a handle on things come the new year? And if you do, how much damage will you have already wrought upon yourself?

Make a Conscious Choice

Think it through. How will the scales of injustice register postholiday? Up, down, sideways? Do you want to lose weight? Maintain? Is it okay to gain a pound or two? There's no right or wrong answer. It's your choice.

Face the Food, Head On

Whether you are trying to lose weight, maintain, or just stay healthy, to get you through this holiday season Our Lady wants you to keep her Top Ten Holiday Commandments in mind. Feel free to copy them and carry them with you. Sometimes a simple reminder is all you need.

The Our Lady of Weight Loss
Top Ten Holiday Commandments

1. **Thou shalt honor thy body and believe in thyself.**
   Be kind, loving, and forgiving to yourself, first and foremost—always.

2. **Thou shalt never leave home hungry.**
   Eat something before the party. A salad, some fruit, even an egg will do. And plenty of water and/or seltzer.

3. **Thou shalt stay clear of the buffet table.**
   Get away from the food. Why torture yourself? Socialize—have a fun conversation!

4. **Thou shalt not deny thyself a treat or two now and then.**
   Fill up your plate with Our Lady–approved foods, and leave a little space for your favorite treat. Too much denial isn't a good thing.

5. **Thou shalt recycle food gifts.**
   Quick, fast—before you change your mind. Give the candy, the cakes, and all red-light, binge-inducing foods away.

6. **Thou shalt keep thy hands busy.**
   Try knitting, crocheting, cutting and pasting, needlepoint, drawing, writing—anything to keep your hands busy. Give your creations as gifts!

7. **Thou shalt stay clear of sweatpants.**
   Wear snug clothing. No room for expansion, no sweats please!

8. **Thou shalt walk—a lot!**
   Ask Santa for a pedometer for Christmas. And then use it!

9. **Thou shalt live in a no-alcohol zone throughout the holidays, so thou doth not lose control.**

10. **Thou shalt not covet thy neighbor's ultra-thin body and ability to eat endlessly without gaining a single ounce.**

Dear Our Lady of Weight Loss,

I love my family. I really do. But family gatherings—in particular, during the holidays—do me in. Everyone expresses love through food. Sometimes it takes weeks to recover, and by the time I come out of my food fog, I've gained a minimum of six pounds. I'd really like to make this year different. Any suggestions?
~Fond of My Family . . . But!

Dear Fond of My Family . . . ,

If you want this year to be different than any other, you'll need to shift the focus from food to fun. Try one of the following things to do at family gatherings. Be creative!

- Bring a camera and really get into it. When Aunt Sue tells Uncle Mike that he's had too much stuffing, snap it!
- Group activities are always fun. How about a game of cards? Or a big jigsaw puzzle spilled on a table, and people can rotate whenever they like. It's a great no-food zone.
- If you anticipate needing some quiet time, instead of bringing the crudités or fruit platter already made, bring all the pieces in a bag, sequester yourself in the kitchen, and cut away. Take your time. Make the platter gorgeous. (Then photograph it.)
- If your parents or grandparents are there, interview them and get them to tell their stories, things you've never heard before—things you've been wondering about.
- Dance. Sing. Tell jokes.
- Bring your knitting, crocheting, cross-stitching. Keep your hands and mind occupied and calm.
- Organize a goofy grab bag gift exchange. That's always good for a few laughs.

I hope that's helpful. ~ Our Lady of Weight Loss

Pious Project
FOTO FOOD JOURNAL

Food journaling keeps us honest. It helps us keep track of what we eat and identify when and why we eat. In other words, it can shed light on our eating habits, and statistics show that those who keep food journals are more successful at losing weight and keeping it off than those who do not.

A picture is worth a thousand words. I wondered how illuminating it might be if I photographed everything (and I mean everything) that I ate. From full-course meals to bites, licks, and tastes. Would I eat less?

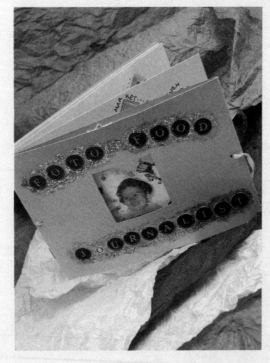

Be more honest? Gain a different kind of insight that journal writing doesn't provide?

What did I learn about myself, and my (dysfunctional) relationship with food? Plenty!

1. I am always eating on the run and out of containers.
2. My bagels are large . . . more than one serving each.
3. I am guilty of multitasking. You know, eating and reading; eating and watching television; eating and talking on the phone.
4. I eat little bits all day long. (I took over a dozen photos in one day!)
5. I love being a foto food journalist! (Should I keep my day job?)

Bottom line: I need to slow down. Maybe this foto food journaling is the answer. Leave it to Our Lady to come up with something so clever!

What to Do?

This week, I'm going to set the table, eat, and only eat—no more multitasking for me. I'm going to eat slowly and savor every bite. And take more photos! Wish me luck.

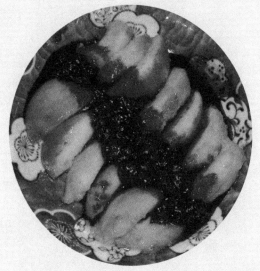

SUPPLIES

One camera. Digital, disposable, or analog (the old-fashioned kind).
Food!

INSTRUCTIONS

Photograph everything you eat. Don't concern yourself with what other people think. If you're out with friends or at an important business meeting, I'm sure all will be impressed with your artistic nature! Just tell them, "I'm a foto food journalist."

When you get the photos back from the lab, or load them onto your computer, take a good look and make a list of things that you've learned about yourself. Were you surprised to see how healthy your eating habits are? Or are there some habits that you might want to work on?

Print and put in your own foto food journalist book! Above all, just plain have fun. Shoot away.

Prickly Prayer

May this year's resolution,
unlike previous resolutions,
stick—like crazy glue.

May this year be the year
that I bid my excess poundage
a fond and final farewell.

May this year be the year
that my fat cells pack their bags and go
by way of the superhighway
to the fat farm in the sky.

As I wave and bid them adieu.

Amen.

Our Lady Jumps Back on the (Resolution) Wagon

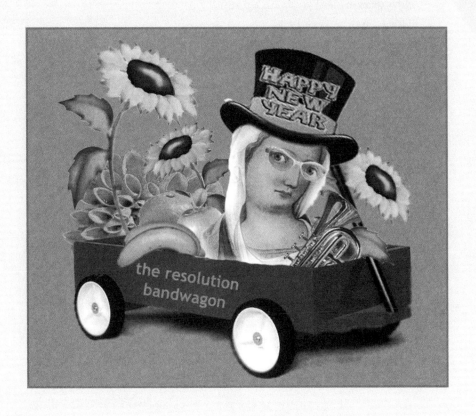

"Resolve to
be thyself;
and know, that he
who finds himself,
loses his misery."
~Matthew Arnold

faᴛoid

Eating long noodles on
the Chinese new year
symbolizes longevity.

MOTIVATIONAL MUSING
Climb Aboard

The Weight-Loss Resolution Bandwagon is leaving the weigh-in station in five minutes.

Did you fall off the proverbial weight-loss bandwagon this holiday season? Did you gain a pound, two, or maybe even four? More?

Not to worry. Weight loss is a process. It requires work, it involves challenges, and falling off the wagon and finding yourself a bit bruised and bloated is par for the course.

Those who reach their weight-loss goals are the ones who get back on the wagon again and again. They learn to see that these setbacks are temporary lapses, and they learn from them. They look at the big picture over a long period of time. They understand that there are no magic bullets, no quick fixes. The turtle wins this race.

Here are a few thoughts and tips to get you and keep you on track.

Practice loving-kindness. Please stop saying mean things to yourself and being so hard on yourself. (If someone else called you a fat pig, you'd punch them in the nose.)

Forgive and forget. Confess your food sins to Our Lady of Weight Loss and move on.

Surrender. Take each day as it comes. Don't put a time limit on your weight-loss goals. As long as you are truly committed to your plan—to yourself—then you are on the right track and you are succeeding.

Postcards from the edge: Buy a pack of postcards or greeting cards, and mail yourself a kind and encouraging note. Getting mail is so much fun. It's okay to be quirky, kooky, and creative when it comes to weight loss. "Hi Jane, I know how hard it was for you to say no to that cake. Bravo and thanks. Love, Jane"

Get support from friends and family or someone who will cheer you on. Steer clear of the saboteurs. (The Our Lady of Weight Loss cheerleaders are here for you. There may even be a Kick in the Tush Club in your neighborhood. Check Our Lady's listings on her Web site—www.ourladyofweightloss.com.)

Positive self-talk. If you think you're not going to make it, you won't. Counter the negative thoughts with positive thoughts: "Yes, I can do this. Losing weight is a piece of cake."

Out with the old. Toss out the devil food, if you please, and stock your house with the right stuff. Do the cleansing ritual (page 23) again and start afresh.

Write out your list of reasons. I want to lose weight because _____. (Fill in the blank, and be honest.) "Be healthy. Look younger. Be socially acceptable. Make that rat who left me feel real bad."

Up your fruit and vegetable intake. "They" recommend eating at least nine servings of fruits and vegetables per day. Remember, you don't want to feel hungry. Fruits and vegetables are vitamin-rich foods that boost your fiber and antioxidant intake and help you feel full.

The 80/20 rule. No one is perfect 100 percent of the time. Not even Our Lady of Weight Loss! If you follow your weight-loss plan 80 percent of the time, and treat yourself to an occasional treat 20 percent of the time, you should be able to achieve and maintain your weight-loss goals.

Practice gratitude. Our Lady of the Gratitude Girdle encourages you to keep a gratitude journal (page 248). Every night before you go to sleep jot down at least five things that you have to be grateful for. Eating is often about filling a void. Perhaps the void isn't as deep as you think!

WEIGHTY CONFESSION

Forgive Me for I Have Sinned

I woke up with a killer headache. For whatever reason, I stumbled into the kitchen for relief (aspirin and food, a weighty combo). There it was—the challah bread that my friend brought to dinner. I should have sent it home with her, because at 5:00 A.M. this morning, banging head in one hand, knife in the other, cutting, I managed to down half a loaf. Did my headache go away? Yes! Was my cure from the bread or the aspirin? Rhetorical question. I am moving on!

All Is Forgiven.
Move On.

Back-on-the-Bandwagon Baked Beans

Ingredients

3 turkey bacon strips

1 tsp. olive oil

$\frac{1}{2}$ cup diced shallots

2 garlic cloves, diced

1 Tbs. chile powder

1 Tbs. ground cumin

1 $14\frac{1}{2}$- oz. can diced
   tomatoes with olive oil
   and red wine flavor

1 $14\frac{1}{2}$-oz. can pinto
   beans, drained

1 $14\frac{1}{2}$-oz. can red kidney
   beans, drained

2 Tbs. hot sauce, smoky flavor
   (I love chipotle sauce.)

$\frac{1}{2}$ cup light brown sugar

$\frac{1}{2}$ to $\frac{3}{4}$ cup water

1 Tbs. cider vinegar

salt and pepper to taste

Directions

Cook turkey bacon as directed on the package.

In a large pot, combine olive oil, shallots, and garlic; cook on medium heat until shallots are soft (about 3 to 5 minutes).

Crumble cooked turkey bacon; add with remaining ingredients.

Bring to boil and then simmer for 45 to 50 minutes, stirring occasionally.

Dishes like this are always better the second day. So I make a pot, let it cool, stick it in the fridge, and reheat it the following day.

Nutrition Facts

Serving Size (287g)
Servings Per Container 6

Amount Per Serving

Calories 260   Calories from Fat 45

	% Daily Value*
Total Fat 5g	8%
Saturated Fat 1g	5%
Trans Fat 0g	
Cholesterol 15mg	5%
Sodium 650mg	27%
Total Carbohydrate 41g	14%
Dietary Fiber 10g	40%
Sugars 15g	
Protein 13g	

Vitamin A 15%	•	Vitamin C 25%
Calcium 10%	•	Iron 25%

*Percent Daily Values are based on a 2,000 calorie diet. Your daily values may be higher or lower depending on your calorie needs:

	Calories	2,000	2,500
Total Fat	Less Than	65g	80g
Saturated Fat	Less Than	20g	25g
Cholesterol	Less Than	300mg	300 mg
Sodium	Less Than	2,400mg	2,400mg
Total Carbohydrate		300g	375g
Dietary Fiber		25g	30g

Calories per gram:
   Fat 9 • Carbohydrate 4 • Protein 4

Our Lady Says You May Never Lick Cake

"I am putting real
plums into an
imaginary cake."
~Mary McCarthy

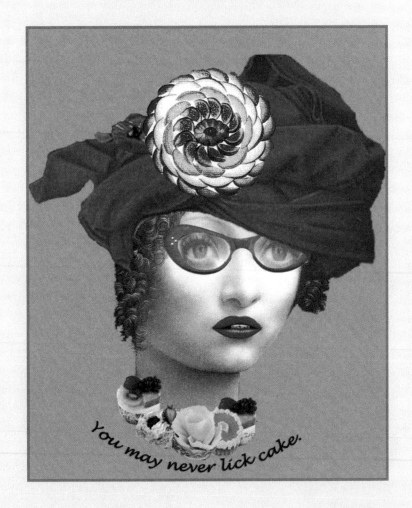

You may never lick cake.

fa T oid

Sugar is actually
sunlight captured and
created by plants during
the process of
photosynthesis and
stored for energy.

MOTIVATIONAL MUSING

Will the Real Cookie Monster Please Stand Up?

Have you made giving up sugar your new year's resolution year after year? Have you tried giving up the three Cs (cookies, cakes, and candy) for Lent? Were you upended by a deep and inexplicable craving for caramel Dulce de Leche Häagen-Dazs ice cream? Are you a sugar addict?

Sugar addiction is no joke. For many years, researchers and doctors did not believe that you could get hooked on an innocent piece of candy or sugar-filled cookie, but now studies that scientists have been compiling over the years suggest sugar addiction may be very real. Certain foods trigger the release of opiate chemicals in the brain.

While it is true that chocolate cheese cake is not in the same league as heroin, alcohol, or nicotine, it appears that some brain responses may be similar. All of these addictions produce a (temporary) pleasurable response that fuels a desire for more. Can you stop at just one chocolate chip double-fudge cookie supreme? I didn't think so.

Did you know that sugar addicts tend to be depleted of key vitamins and minerals, which may weaken their immune systems? The average American consumes approximately twenty-four teaspoons of sugar each day. What's your intake? How much of an addict are you? Do you want to get off the stuff? Confess now!

Here are a few Our Lady of Weight Loss–approved suggestions to help you bust your sugar habit:

Never skip breakfast. (See Our Lady of the Good Morning Meal, page 38.) Those who eat breakfast are less likely to crave sugar. Your body wants that energy boost first thing in the morning to get all your gears in motion. If you skip your morning oatmeal, you're likely to start craving that chocolate chip cookie come afternoon. Low-sugar breakfasts include eggs, whole-grain unsweetened cereal, fruit, and unsweetened yogurt.

Never skip any meal! Skipping meals in general is a bad idea. Eating balanced meals at regular intervals keeps your brain and body fueled, so you don't crave heavy starch or sugar foods for energy.

Get enough sleep. Rest. (See Our Lady of the Sacred Snooze, page 105.) Once again, the body starts to crave starchy and/or sugary food for energy—for fuel. When you feel the need to nap, do so. Listen to your body.

Excessive salt can trigger sugar cravings. Fast-food restaurants and processed foods use salt to stimulate your appetite. They want you to eat more! And be sure to read labels. I did a little pantry reading this morning. I was floored. My husband had to get out the smelling salts. Make low-sodium choices.

Eat whole foods (not refined carbohydrates). Refined, aka empty calorie, foods such as white bread, cookies, cake, and candy don't satisfy your body because they lack nutrients and fiber. Try eating more fruit, carrots, beets, sweet potatoes, winter squash. They're loaded with the good stuff.

And sorry to say: there's no donut in the world that's going to take away your emotional pulls and pain. Try yoga, walking, or talking to a friend.

I know—easier said than done—but no one said bustin' sugar would be easy.

Dear Our Lady of Weight Loss,

I just can't seem to lick my sugar addiction. Should I check myself into the Betty Ford clinic? Help! ~Hooked

Dear Hooked,

It may seem like a losing battle, but hang in there. You can do it. Trying eating fruits and high-sugar vegetables like carrots, beets, and winter squash. The more whole foods you eat, the less likely you are to give in to your addiction. And try picking up a crochet hook! Keep you hands and mind busy. We're rootin' for you. ~Our Lady of Weight Loss

Pious Project

I have a long history with cake. When I was a child, the names Betty Crocker and Sara Lee were bandied about at home with such frequency that I began to think of them as family members. My mother taught me that it was a sin to put the cake away if the edges weren't straight. But when she tried to cut a straight piece, somehow or other the edges were left jagged. We'd have to cut another and yet another piece of cake to "even" it—sometimes until the entire cake was gone. "Thankfully," she told me, "there are no calories in jagged pieces."

Since cake is inexorably a part of my childhood landscape, there's no way I'm giving it up. I am willing, however, to change my relationship with it. So instead of eating cake, I now sew myself a piece. It's twenty times as satisfying—no kidding. And everlasting, too!

SUPPLIES

1 delicious picture of your favorite cake (4" x 6")
1 sheet of computer transfer paper (for light or white material)
1 piece of white or off-white fabric—cotton, silk, or satin
iron
1 piece of 4" x 6" watercolor paper
sewing machine (hand sew)
thread (pretty colors of your choice)
pillow stuffing (available at sewing supply store)

Note: You will need a computer and printer for this, or you can take your photo and transfer paper to the local copy store.

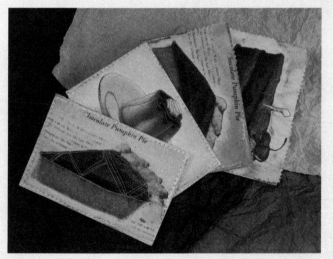

INSTRUCTIONS

Print your delicious cake picture on computer transfer paper. (Follow printing instructions on transfer paper package.)

Heat transfer (fancy way of saying iron) image onto fabric.

Trim fabric to fit 4" x 6" piece of watercolor paper.

Sew image to watercolor paper, leaving opening large enough to stuff (with pillow stuffing). Caution: Don't overstuff.

Sew closed.

And *now* comes the fun part. Follow the lines of the cake with your thread. Change colors, try zigzags, get into it. Experience the icing as lines, swirls, colors. Cake as art—yum!

Prickly Prayer

Dear Our Lady of Holy Water,

Please may I thirst for water
and experience with every sip
its miraculous cleansing powers.

May my sins as well as fat be washed away
and permanently eliminated from my body.

And please,
May there always be a clean bathroom nearby.

Amen.

Kick No. 24

Our Lady of Holy Water

"Beware of those
who stir the
waters to pretend
they are deep."
~Chinese proverb

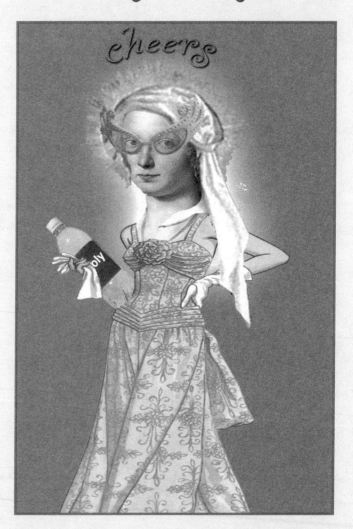

fa T oid

Most of the world's people must walk at least three hours to fetch water.

MOTIVATIONAL MUSING

Cheers!

Water, a holy life force, is the most plentiful liquid on earth. Water covers approximately 70 percent of the earth's surface and is an essential component in most living things. Our bodies are more than 75 percent water, our blood more than 80 percent, our muscles more than 75 percent and our brains more than 76 percent.

Water regulates the temperature of the human body. It carries nutrients and oxygen to cells, cushions joints, and protects organs and tissues.

Water can help to alleviate depression, cleanse impurities from the body, and make our largest organ—our skin—glow with health.

Water is a natural lubricant. It helps everything slide through your system.

Water fights bad breath.

Water also helps to make us look younger. Skin that is saggy (due to the aging process or weight loss) plumps up beautifully when the skin cells are hydrated.

Water improves muscle tone. Hydrated muscles contract more easily, which makes for a more effective workout.

Water is a natural appetite suppressant and helps us to digest our food. It even promotes weight loss and helps the body to metabolize fat into energy. A recent study found that drinking 17 ounces of water increases your metabolism by 30 percent within ten minutes, and within thirty minutes your metabolism peaks.

And being dehydrated decreases your body's ability to burn calories by 2 percent each day, according to research done at the University of Utah.

How much water should we drink? To stay at a maximum burning level, you should drink approximately eight glasses of water daily, and limit those caffeinated drinks. Your body only absorbs about half of the liquid in soda, juice, and tea, as opposed to two thirds of water.

Water is the most important nutrient. Cheers!

Pious Project

I find it difficult to drink eight glasses of water each and every day, so I start my day by downing two, straight up, upon waking. Of course, this creates other challenges. Should I need to leave my apartment, and should the water have made its way through me before I reach my destination, where might I relieve myself?

To solve this problem, I made a map of my most traveled route, and mapped out all the "public" restrooms. Granted, my friend, June's bathroom isn't public, but she's a kind soul, and if you say "Our Lady of Weight Loss sent me," she'll let you in!

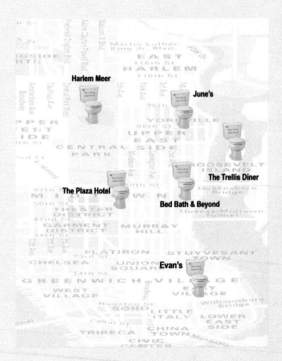

Kick No. 25

Our Lady of Smilology

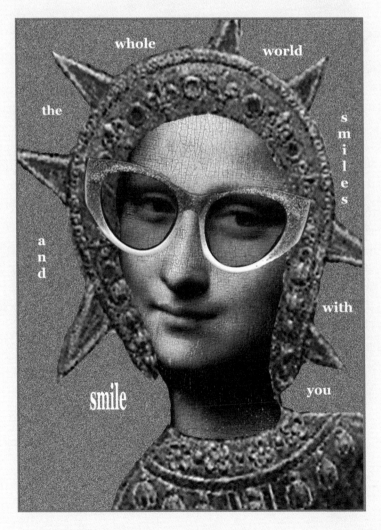

the whole world smiles and smile you with smiles

"There's a smile on my face for the whole human race."
~Alan Jay Lerner

153

faToid

It takes twenty-six
muscles to smile, and
sixty-two to frown.

MOTIVATIONAL MUSING
Smile and Say "Cheese"

One of the best things you can do for yourself and for everyone around you is to smile. Smiling brings oxygen to your brain, makes you feel better immediately, and sends out comforting messages to others. Smiling pulls people in nice and close.

A true smile comes from genuine pleasure. Two sets of facial muscles are used to create this smile. The first set is in the cheeks that pull up the corners of the mouth; the second set is around the eyes. These muscles cause the eyes to narrow and crinkle.

Smiling can make you look like an inviting, accepting, likable, and pleasant person (even if you're not). When you first meet someone, if you don't smile that person is likely to think that you're not interested in or attracted to them. They may even think you are a cold potato. So, even if you're feeling blue or simply not in the mood to smile, do yourself a favor—smile anyway. Fake it until you make it!

The health benefits of smiling are plentiful.

Smiling~
♦ increases the production of endorphins, natural pain killers, and serotonin, a hormone that regulates your mood;
♦ boosts your immune system and increases the number and activity of antibodies that fight infection;
♦ lowers your blood pressure;
♦ helps you to relax;

- relieves stress;
- enhances respiratory function;
- exercises fifteen to twenty-six facial muscles;
- makes you look younger as it lifts the face;
- fires up various parts of the brain!

Tasty Tidbit **More fabulous facts about smiling that are sure to make you grin.**

- Seventy-two percent of people think that those who smile frequently are confident and successful.
- Eighty-six percent of people are more likely to talk to strangers if they are smiling.
- Bosses are 12 percent more likely to promote people who smile a lot.
- Research shows that 65 percent of communication is nonverbal (some say even higher).
- Studies show that happiness is a by-product of smiling, not that those who are happy smile, as most people assume.

The simple act of smiling can change your day.

Say Cheese!

Nutrition Facts

Serving Size 1/4 cup (82g)
Servings Per Container 5

Amount Per Serving

Calories 60	Calories from Fat 0

	% Daily Value*
Total Fat 0g	**0%**
Saturated Fat 0g	**0%**
Trans Fat 0g	
Cholesterol 0mg	**0%**
Sodium 0mg	**0%**
Total Carbohydrate 16g	**5%**
Dietary Fiber 1g	**4%**
Sugars 13g	
Protein 0g	

Vitamin A 0%	•	Vitamin C 15%
Calcium 2%	•	Iron 2%

*Percent Daily Values are based on a 2,000 calorie diet. Your daily values may be higher or lower depending on your calorie needs:

	Calories	2,000	2,500
Total Fat	Less Than	65g	80g
Saturated Fat	Less Than	20g	25g
Cholesterol	Less Than	300mg	300 mg
Sodium	Less Than	2,400mg	2,400mg
Total Carbohydrate		300g	375g
Dietary Fiber		25g	30g

Calories per gram:
Fat 9 • Carbohydrate 4 • Protein 4

RIGHTEOUS RECIPE
Blueberry Sauce

*F*rom Abby, my daughter.

Pour this sauce on your toast or fruit, mix with yogurt, or just eat it by the spoonful. It is divine.

Ingredients

   ¼ cup water
   ¼ cup light brown sugar
   juice from freshly squeezed lemon
   1 pt. of blueberries

Directions

   Heat water with light brown sugar until dissolved. Add lemon juice.

   Then the blueberries. Just keep cookin' and stirrin' until it breaks down and it's all saucy.

✳ **Dear Our Lady of Weight Loss,**
✳ *I tried to dig deep and smile when the receptionist slipped me my weigh-in book*
✳ *at my weekly weight-loss meeting and I noted the 2.8 pound gain. I know there*
✳ *are worse things in life, and that people have real problems (can't think of any*
✳ *right now), but I am filled with despair.* ~Fat and Shallow

Dear Fat and Shallow,

Oh my, you're calling yourself names. Compounding the misery. You are entitled to feel despair. Who isn't when it comes to weight loss or gain? Just don't wallow in it too long. Give yourself a few minutes of self-pity, and then look in the mirror and say with conviction, "I'm back on track. The scale owes me and will deliver next week." Feel better? ~Our Lady of Weight Loss

Pious Project

I've always had this thing for sending and receiving mail—snail mail—the old-fashioned way. You remember, don't you? You use pens, write longhand, put postage stamps on envelopes, walk to a mailbox, and say a send-off prayer as the envelopes make their way down the mail shoot.

Now I make and send Inspiration by Post cards to my friends. It's so much fun!

And sometimes I receive Inspiration by Post cards! My mom sent me this Thinking of You card after I'd lost fifty pounds. We'd had a conversation in which we decided that I had become half my previous size.

Here's how Mom made this card.

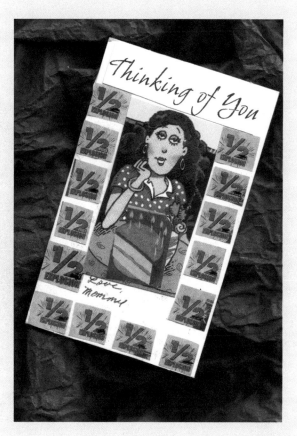

SUPPLIES

old greeting cards
scissors
glue stick
supermarket flyer
pen
postcard postage stamp

INSTRUCTIONS

Cut bits and pieces from old greeting cards (Mom loves to recycle); she cut phrases and photos and pasted them onto a 4" x 6" piece of hard stock (from an old greeting card). She then added a border of $\frac{1}{2}$ explosions that were printed on her local supermarket flyer. And then she signed it lovingly, and put it in the mail.

It was simple, easy, fun, and delighted my soul.

Thanks, Mom

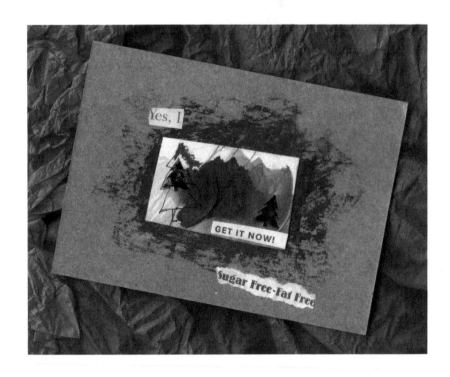

Kick No. 26

Our Lady of Feng Shui Red

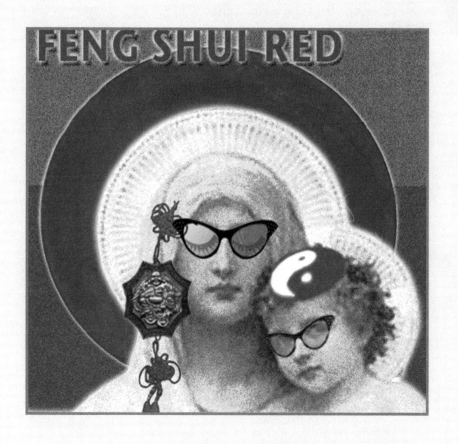

"When in doubt
wear red."
~Bill Blass

faToid

During the Depression restaurant owners found that diners would eat less if the food was served on a blue plate; thus the term "blue plate special."

MOTIVATIONAL MUSING

Feng Shui and the Blue Plate Special

Feng shui (pronounced "fung shway"), the Chinese art of placement, translates literally as "wind water." Wind represents that which we cannot see and water represents that which we cannot grasp. Feng shui helps to harmonize these unseen forces in our lives.

According to ancient Chinese philosophy (and the laws of physics), all things—both living and nonliving—are composed of energy. This energy is called *chi*. It is the life force of all matter. Through the principles of feng shui one can create a balanced and harmonious environment, which in turn creates a happier, healthier, wealthier, better life for you.

Feng shui is used primarily in interior and exterior home design. However, the same principles can give support to those who want to lose weight.

The kitchen, one of the most important rooms for health and wealth, should be organized. Your stove should be kept clean. Your refrigerator and pantry should be stocked with foods that are *not* past their expiration dates! (I'm in violation.) Be sure to place a bowl of fresh fruit on the counter or table. This represents vitality and healthy choices.

Bright-colored foods should be well represented on your plate, while neutral color foods should be less than one third. The chi value in a bowl of veggies far exceeds the chi in a plate of pasta.

Be sure to balance the five elements of feng shui—earth, metal, water, wood, and fire—and yin (alkaline) foods and yang (acid) foods. It's all about resonating with your space. When your chi is up, you feel good, and are less likely to gorge, binge, or go on a bender.

The water element (represented by the colors blue and black) is extremely important, as it will slow down your eating process. Dinnerware should be either black or dark blue. The color of the plate subconsciously affects your appetite. Dark colors diminish your appetite. Bright colors, like red, stimulate your appetite!

Place a dark tablecloth on your table after lunch. Your appetite should lessen as the day progresses. Decorate your table with fresh flowers. Use your best china for all your meals, making eating a sacred ritual.

Aside from the visual effects, let's consider smell and sound. Free-flowing music, such as Gregorian chants or New Age sounds may enable you to slow down and savor your meal. Interesting concept!

For an even more satisfying and sensual experience, consider adding the scent of chamomile or rose oil to the dining table.

WEIGHTY CONFESSION

Forgive Me for I Have Sinned

I finally got a Costco card—walked past all the nuts/candies/ice creams—and then bought a forty-count box of Rice Krispies Treats—my fave.
This is insanity.

All Is Forgiven.
Move On.

Pious Project
LIGHT-SWITCH PLATES

I confess!

I had a dysfunctional relationship with the kitchen. It was always a *red hot zone*. The mere mention of the word and a sugar glaze fell over me.

As it turned out, my kitchen's feng shui was way off. I cleaned everything thoroughly, hung a bamboo mirror on the back wall, placed a gorgeous iron tea kettle on the counter, and then I created these ultra hip and snazzy feng shui light-switch plates.

I thought, what better way to remind me that the kitchen is not the enemy than to make an Our Lady of Feng Shui Red Kitchen Light Switch. It is indeed a fun, happy place that is home to conscious eating.

SUPPLIES

acrylic gesso (Gesso is a primer and it provides "tooth" to the surface of the switch plate so it will hold whatever else you glue or paint on top of it.)

light-switch plate

gel medium, heavy gel gloss (Gel medium acts both as a glue and a shiny varnish. You brush under and over everything! It dries translucent.)

1" foam brushes (at art supply or household paint stores)

words and images from newspapers and/or magazines, or wrapping paper; whatever pleases your palate!

glitter, nail polish, anything that is fun to work with!

INSTRUCTIONS

Gesso the switch plate and let dry.

Using your foam brush and the gel medium, glue bits and pieces of paper to the plate. You are creating a background layer, so feel free to rip and glue without too much thought.

Arrange any photos and/or words on the plate. Really, there's no right or wrong way to do this. Whatever pleases you.

Glue down (using the same brush).

Add a layer or two more of the gel medium on top. It acts as a protective covering and shines a bit while remaining translucent.

My creations included fruit wrapping paper (see the mango, kiwi, and bananas?), as well as red glitter.

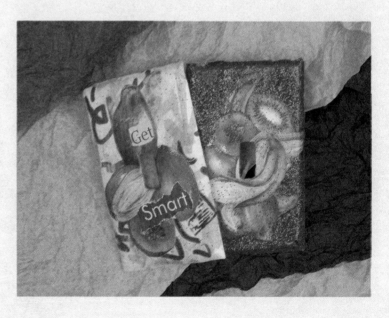

Our Lady of Creative Acts of Weight Loss

"If you hear a
voice within you
say 'you cannot
paint,' then by all
means paint, and
that voice will
be silenced."

~Vincent van Gogh

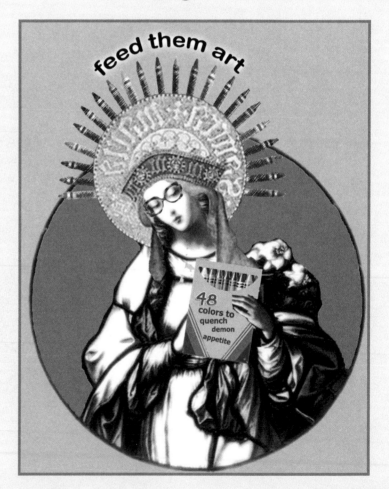

feed them art

48
colors to
quench
demon
appetite

faⓉoid

The average adult
thinks of three to six
alternative ways to sort
out any given situation.
The average child
thinks of sixty.

MOTIVATIONAL MUSING

What Is a Creative Act of Weight Loss?

A creative act of weight loss is something we do that is considered innovative and/or productive, in place of answering the call to eat when not hungry.

Dear Our Lady of Weight Loss,

Boredom. Anger. Happiness. Sadness. Loneliness. Frustration. Anxiety. They all screamed to be fed. But I faced them head on.

"What do you want?" I asked.

"Chocolate," cried Boredom.

"Lemon," said Anger.

"Carrot cake for me, please," sobbed Sadness.

I made each demon a cupcake to his liking. "These sweets are ever-lasting," I told them.

After crocheting for hours and hours, concentrating on the texture, the line, the color of the cupcake—not the taste—I realized that I had committed a creative act of weight loss! My relationship with the cup-cake family is forever changed.

Thanks for the new perspective. ~Cupcake Crocheter

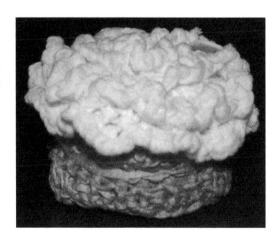

Intellectually, we know that food is just food, but over the decades of overeating we have given it a great deal of power. Some of us think about food all the time.

Committing creative acts of weight loss present opportunities to stare down the enemy and allow our creativity to surface. We're taking a leap of faith into an adventure that can lead us out of the dark forest of dieting, regaining, bingeing, and purging, into the light of creation.

Who Is Creative?

There are plenty of ways to be creative, and the truth is—yes, you are creative. (When you made breakfast this morning, Did you create a healthy start to the day? Or did you create a donut-filled sugar rush–filled morning?)

Research shows that any person of average intelligence or aptitude is capable of committing creative acts of weight loss.

Your creativity is shaped by your experiences, your talent (yes, you are naturally loaded with it), your ability to think and approach subjects in new ways (looking at weight loss from a new angle, as in, weight loss is fun), and your capacity to push through despite missteps, mishaps, and slipups (it's not hopeless, no matter how many times you have failed; it's just part of the process).

Be excited. You're on the road to Sveltesville. Yahoooo! Enthusiasm will give you a creative boost and you will approach weight loss naturally, with an open mind and from a more positive and creative place. Our Lady of Weight Loss is convinced that vast creative resources lie dormant within you. You can realize your potential. You can integrate the essence of who you are—your thinner core—into your weight-loss plan.

Knock down those self-imposed "I can't do this, this is too hard" barriers! Be creative about your weight-loss plan.

Plunge right in. There are plenty of pious projects throughout this book that can help you change your relationship with food. Get goin'!

Tasty Tidbit Here are some ways to help get your creative juices flowing (and to keep you out of the kitchen).

Listen to Bach. The consensus of opinion is that listening to music by Johann Sebastian Bach can get your creative genius flowing. It's certainly worth a try.

Keep a journal. Writing down your thoughts can loosen up those blocks.

Take a walk. Walking/moving always gives my genius a boost.

Deep breathing. Getting oxygen to the brain is always a good idea.

Change your routine. Take a new route to work, listen to a new radio station, read a comic book.

Note: I did not say to watch a new television show.

Be inspired. Read about your favorite genius: Albert Einstein, Helen Keller, Eleanor Roosevelt.

WEIGHTY
CONFESSION
Forgive Me for I Have Sinned

I just ate *tacos* for the first time in probably fifteen years. I had my dog Bob at work with me today and was trying to think of something I could eat that wouldn't involve leaving him in the hot car while I ran into the store. And some other people walked by my office talking about Taco Tuesday, so I went for it. But . . . I feel like a grotesque now. Why did I do that? I don't even eat meat but about four times a year. I'm polluted. Forgive me for I have sinned.

All Is Forgiven.

Move On.

From Josh, my son!

Ingredients

4 cloves of garlic, smashed and chopped coarsely

1 Tbs. olive oil (two if you want to splurge)

1 yellow juicy tomato, sliced thin

salt and pepper to taste

nonstick spray

2 whole wheat tortillas

cayenne pepper

¼ cup chopped cilantro

Directions

Preheat oven to about 450°.

Mix garlic with a tablespoon or two of olive oil.

Slice one tomato (yellow, if available) and mix with oil, salt, and pepper to taste.

Lightly oil (or spray) a baking sheet and place tortillas, lightly sprinkled with cayenne.

Arrange tomato slices on the tortillas and top with a couple of sprigs of coarsely chopped cilantro.

Bake for 15 minutes, or until tortillas are browned and crispy.

Nutrition Facts

Serving Size (78g)
Servings Per Container 4

Amount Per Serving

Calories 90   Calories from Fat 35

		% Daily Value*
Total Fat 4g		6%
Saturated Fat 0g		0%
Trans Fat 0g		
Cholesterol 0mg		0%
Sodium 30mg		1%
Total Carbohydrate 11g		4%
Dietary Fiber 1g		4%
Sugars 2g		
Protein 3g		

Vitamin A 8%	•	Vitamin C 20%
Calcium 2%	•	Iron 2%

*Percent Daily Values are based on a 2,000 calorie diet. Your daily values may be higher or lower depending on your calorie needs:

	Calories	2,000	2,500
Total Fat	Less Than	65g	80g
Saturated Fat	Less Than	20g	25g
Cholesterol	Less Than	300mg	300 mg
Sodium	Less Than	2,400mg	2,400mg
Total Carbohydrate		300g	375g
Dietary Fiber		25g	30g

Calories per gram:
Fat 9 • Carbohydrate 4 • Protein 4

Our Lady of Deep-Seated Beliefs

"You will never be happier than you expect. To change your happiness, change your expectation."

~Bette Davis

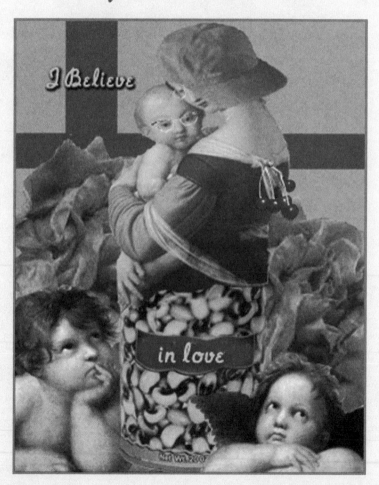

MOTIVATIONAL MUSING
A Penny to Change Your Thoughts

faToid

Ninety-five percent
of what we know about
the brain is based on
information learned in
the last twenty years.
Many of your beliefs
were more than
likely shaped by
erroneous information.

What is a belief system? A belief system is a series of ideas that your mind has organized in order to project an image of what is real. It encompasses everything you think about yourself, others, and the world at large. It is filled with should haves and ought tos.

Our beliefs are formed throughout our childhoods and come from our interactions with others, such as our parents, friends, teachers, institutions, newspapers, television, etc. They are generally acted out in adulthood without much thought or examination.

These systems are mighty powerful, and they have a profound impact on the ways in which we lead our lives. Our beliefs tell us how to feel and behave, and they provide the foundation from which we approach the world.

If we do not challenge our belief systems, they will remain unchanged. You may find that some of your beliefs are empowering. Great! Keep those beliefs and build on them. It's the outdated and limiting beliefs that are in need of an overhaul!

Your belief about your ability to lose weight and keep it off strongly influences your internal dialogue, which, in turn, strongly influences your choices.

Do you believe that you are in control of your weight loss? Or do you believe that some alien force has taken control and force-fed you?

Do you believe that you can set realistic, measurable goals and achieve them, no matter what? Or, do you believe that when things aren't going your way, when you're having a bad day, you're just gonna have to eat?

Do you believe that you can lose weight and keep it off? Or, do you believe that all those photos of your heavy relatives determine your weight and size?

Do you believe that your past attempts at weight loss were learning experiences, and that those who are successful are often not successful the first time out? Or, do you believe that your inability to lose and keep off those extra pounds is a sign that you are a loser (the "bad" kind of loser) and that you are doomed?

Do you believe that you are really buying those cookies for the kids? (Oh, come on!)

Food for thought: What are your weight loss beliefs? What set of guiding principles do you believe to be true about yourself? Where or from whom did they come? How can you change them and yourself? Awareness is the first step.

Tasty Tidbit **Take Five**

According to researchers at the Oregon Health Sciences University, women who do absolutely nothing for five minutes each day are more likely to lose weight than those who don't take time to relax. Those stress hormones, which increase appetite, will get you every time!

RIGHTEOUS RECIPE
Krispy Kale

Hails from Mary Margaret of Houston, Texas.

"Dark green kale has more nutrients than any other vegetable," says Mary Margaret. She says that a good way to eat an entire bunch of kale is to tear it into bite-size pieces and put on a sprayed (with olive oil or nonstick spray) cookie (pardon the expression) sheet. Dust with Parmesan cheese and put under the broiler for a very short time, until crispy. "I eat all those vitamins right off the tray by the stove," she says. "It never gets to the table. Feels absolutely virtuous."

Ingredients

8 cups kale

nonstick spray

4 Tbs. grated Parmesan cheese

1 tsp. curry powder

$\frac{1}{2}$ cup chopped pecans or slivered almonds

Directions

Preheat oven to 400°.

Stir all ingredients except nuts until well blended and place on the cookie sheet. Scatter the nuts over the top.

Broil for 2 to 3 minutes.

Serve at once.

Nutrition Facts		
Serving Size (79g)		
Servings Per Container 8		
Amount Per Serving		
Calories 100	Calories from Fat 60	
		% Daily Value*
Total Fat 7g		11%
Saturated Fat 1.5g		8%
Trans Fat 0g		
Cholesterol 5mg		2%
Sodium 80mg		3%
Total Carbohydrate 8g		3%
Dietary Fiber 2g		8%
Sugars 0g		
Protein 4g		
Vitamin A 210% • Vitamin C 130%		
Calcium 15% • Iron 8%		

*Percent Daily Values are based on a 2,000 calorie diet. Your daily values may be higher or lower depending on your calorie needs:

	Calories	2,000	2,500
Total Fat	Less Than	65g	80g
Saturated Fat	Less Than	20g	25g
Cholesterol	Less Than	300mg	300 mg
Sodium	Less Than	2,400mg	2,400mg
Total Carbohydrate		300g	375g
Dietary Fiber		25g	30g

Calories per gram:
Fat 9 • Carbohydrate 4 • Protein 4

WEIGHTY CONFESSION

Forgive Me for I Have Sinned

The day after the pope died, short of sleep and suffocating in grief, I grabbed a large bag of BBQ Fritos and downed the whole bag in less than three minutes. Wash away my sin and the yellow number 5 dye.

All Is Forgiven.

Move On.

Pious Project

A HEART FULL OF ART

Sometimes we feel empty and fill ourselves with food instead of love, life, and/or art.

When I'm feeling empty, I make heart postcards and salt them away in this box. When my heart is brimming over with art, I mail a card or two to friends.

You can fill your Heart Full of Art with anything that makes you feel full: family photos, homemade cards, souvenirs from trips. What makes your heart sing?

SUPPLIES

2 sponge brushes (one for paint, one for glue)
1 heart-shaped box
red acrylic paint
rice paper

craft glue
orange acrylic paint
heart-shape stencils
silver glass beads
tassel trim

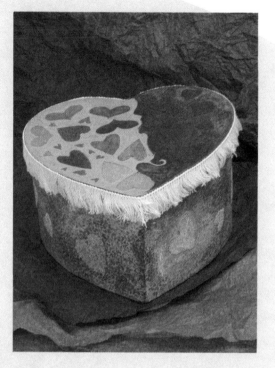

INSTRUCTIONS

Using your sponge brush, paint your heart-shaped box with a coat of red paint.

Rip up a bunch of rice paper (white or any color that you may be thirsting for) into pieces from 1" to 3" in length.

With sponge brush, using craft glue, cover the box with these ripped pieces. Overlapping is fine. Rice paper is fabulous. It melts into the box and leaves a subtle layer of color and pattern.

Smear a little orange paint on the brush and spread a light coat over the rice paper. Sometimes I do a good job of cleaning my brush in between colors, and sometimes not. I actually prefer when there's a little of the first color left. It makes for interesting and unpredictable streaks. Art surprises and happy accidents are the best.

Adhere another layer of rice paper with craft glue (both undercoat and overcoat).

When dry, I stencil hearts on the box. I know that a heart shape is easy enough to sketch, but if you want them to be uniform in size and shape, it's best to use a stencil. Then I paint the hearts with red or orange paint.

Paint some craft glue in the hearts and sprinkle with silver glass beads.

For a nice finishing touch, glue a tassel trim around the rim.

Our Lady of the High-Calorie Burn

"Cigarette sales would drop to zero overnight if the warning said, 'Cigarettes Contain Fat.'"
~Dave Barry

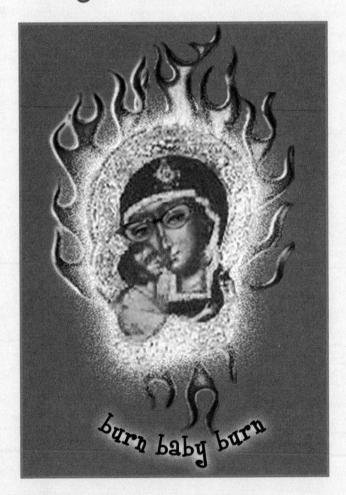

MOTIVATIONAL MUSING
What Is a Calorie?

I queried my posse of nutrition-minded friends. "What is a calorie?"

While most people know what a calorie does—gives us energy, fuels us, and sometimes if we eat foods that have too many of them, adds weight to our bodies—they're not exactly sure how to define it.

A calorie is a unit of heat. It is the amount of heat required to raise the temperature of one gram of water one degree Celsius. All calories come from either carbohydrates, proteins, fats, or alcohol.

- Each gram of carbs contains 3.75 calories.
- Each gram of fat contains 9 calories.
- Each gram of protein contains 4 calories.
- Each gram of alcohol contains 7 calories.

Most of us think of calories in relation to food (and weight), as in, "This piece of cake has 540 calories. I'll blow my entire day if I eat this."

A calorie is also a unit of measurement of energy produced by food when it is used in the body. We need calories to fuel us. If we ingest more fuel into our bodies than we need for the amount of activity we do, our bodies will store this unused fuel. It may be stored as fat, or as muscle, if we perform enough muscle-building exercises (i.e., weight lifting).

Bottom Line

It's a simple matter of calories in and calories burned. You burn calories (fuel) when you perform physical activities, and you also burn calories just by sitting still, breathing, and even thinking. A person who is physically active can eat more calories each day without gaining weight, because this person is using the fuel she pumps into her body, rather than storing it! If you eat more calories than you burn, you will gain weight.

Dear Our Lady of Weight Loss,

Please enroll me in your Kick in the Tush. Please be gentle, as my tush is sensitive from squeezing my glutes at the gym. I did six pull-ups the other day, and although there were only five people in the gym at the time, everybody stopped what they were doing and cheered me on. It was such an awesome, supportive feeling. I would also like to point out that I have to reach all the way up while standing on my toes to even reach the pull-up bar. Even as recently as three months ago I would not have thought this possible. My next goal is to get my bicycle fixed and be able to ride my five-mile morning walk. I'll keep you posted. I am putting your Web site in my Favorites. ~Steve E., Petaluma, California

Dear Steve E.

Thanks much for the delightful letter. Not only did it make me laugh—it sent me straight to the gym! I hope others will be inspired by your note. We all need to cheer each other on. Go Steve-e; go Steve-e. Go!!!
~Our Lady of Weight Loss

Kick 'em and Twist 'em:
Exercise Tips for Exercise Flunkies

1. Pretend you're Madonna: Blast the music and dance in your underwear (when no one's home, of course).
2. Remember the hula hoop? Let's start it up again! Why not?
3. Hopscotch was the one and only game I could play when I was a kid. Grab some chalk, your kid or your neighbor's, and hit the sidewalks.
4. Walk backward. It works an entirely different set of muscles. And makes you laugh!
5. Twister. Twist away with your partner and end the night in a heated sweat.

RIGHTEOUS RECIPE
Amilah's Fruit Tootin' Smoothie

This smoothie is from Amilah, Chicago.

To be sure you can make this smoothie at any time:

- Always keep a supply of cleaned organic strawberries or blueberries, along with bananas cut in thirds, in the freezer.
- Always keep a bottle of (no sugar added) tangy special fruit juice (e.g., blueberry or pomegranate) in the fridge.
- Always keep either low-fat yogurt or soy yogurt around— in good flavors. (Peach is always good in the mix.)

Nutrition Facts

Serving Size (284g)
Servings Per Container

Amount Per Serving

Calories 180	Calories from Fat 10

% Daily Value*

Total Fat 1g	**2%**
Saturated Fat 0g	**0%**
Trans Fat 0g	
Cholesterol 5mg	**2%**
Sodium 35mg	**1%**
Total Carbohydrate 40g	**13%**
Dietary Fiber 4g	**16%**
Sugars 27g	
Protein 4g	

Vitamin A 2%	•	Vitamin C 25%	
Calcium 8%	•	Iron 4%	

*Percent Daily Values are based on a 2,000 calorie diet. Your daily values may be higher or lower depending on your calorie needs:

		Calories	2,000	2,500
Total Fat	Less Than		65g	80g
Saturated Fat	Less Than		20g	25g
Cholesterol	Less Than		300mg	300 mg
Sodium	Less Than		2,400mg	2,400mg
Total Carbohydrate			300g	375g
Dietary Fiber			25g	30g

Calories per gram:
Fat 9 • Carbohydrate 4 • Protein 4

Directions

When the smoothie bug hits, get the blender and the equivalent of one banana and $1\frac{1}{2}$ cups of berries per banana per person. Add $\frac{1}{2}$ to 1 cup of that special juice, scoop in the yogurt, and fill to above the frozen fruit line with cold filtered water.

Blend.

Serve in a glass with a straw.

Yum. Easy.

And truly, there's no need for honey or extra sweeteners—the banana makes it way sweet.

Our Lady of the Fidgety Few

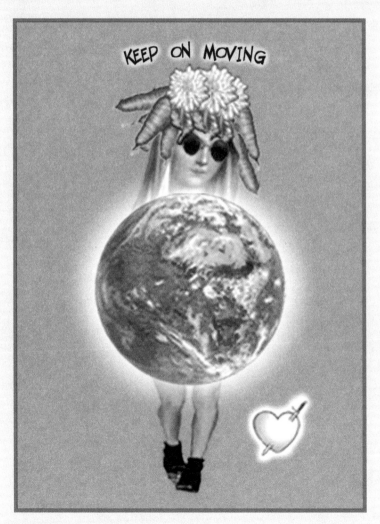

"I feel about
exercise the same
way that I feel
about a few
other things:
that there is
nothing wrong
with it if it is
done in private
by consenting
adults."
~Anna Quindlen

faToid

Your muscles do not
grow during exercise.
Exercise is the stimulus.
Your body strengthens
its muscles while
you are resting.

MOTIVATIONAL MUSING
Move Your Bloomin' Arse

The Mayo clinic found that fidgety people are thinner than those who just sit. In fact, those who were seated for an average of 150 minutes more a day than their squirmy counterparts burned 350 fewer calories per day!

The restless, by the way, didn't spend their time at the gym. No, they were tapping their feet, as well as shopping, cleaning, running errands, and playing music and making art!

Want to join the ranks of the squirmy and restless? Tap, wiggle, and squirm, whenever possible.

Those who exercise at least three and a half hours per week are 25 percent to 30 percent less likely to die prematurely!

And for young and old alike, exercise helps you maintain healthy bones, muscles, and joints and keeps you steady on your feet, so you are less likely to fall!

Research shows that three ten-minute periods of exercise can be just as or possibly more effective than one thirty-minute period. You might want to consider three different segments: one for the upper body, one for the lower body, and finally, the abs!

Tasty Tidbit **Exercise**

lowers your risk for heart disease;

restores function to the heart after an attack;

reduces the risk of developing several cancers, including those of the breast, prostate, and colon;

reduces the risk of developing diabetes;

can significantly lessen feelings of depression and anxiety, and promotes psychological well-being;

helps to control weight;

helps to regulate stress;

keeps your metabolism elevated throughout the day.

RIGHTEOUS RECIPE
Tofu and Zucchini Stir-Fry

Ingredients

couscous

1 10-oz. can of no-fat chicken broth

2 cloves garlic, crushed

1-inch hunk of ginger, grated

6 scallions

2 medium-size zucchinis

1 medium tomato, diced

Nutrition Facts

Serving Size (332g)
Servings Per Container 4

Amount Per Serving

Calories 230   Calories from Fat 70

	% Daily Value*
Total Fat 8g	**12%**
Saturated Fat 1.5g	**8%**
Trans Fat 0g	
Cholesterol 0mg	**0%**
Sodium 450mg	**19%**
Total Carbohydrate 25g	**8%**
Dietary Fiber 4g	**16%**
Sugars 3g	
Protein 19g	

Vitamin A 10%	•	Vitamin C 30%
Calcium 15%	•	Iron 20%

*Percent Daily Values are based on a 2,000 calorie diet. Your daily values may be higher or lower depending on your calorie needs:

	Calories	2,000	2,500
Total Fat	Less Than	65g	80g
Saturated Fat	Less Than	20g	25g
Cholesterol	Less Than	300mg	300 mg
Sodium	Less Than	2,400mg	2,400mg
Total Carbohydrate		300g	375g
Dietary Fiber		25g	30g

Calories per gram:
Fat 9 • Carbohydrate 4 • Protein 4

---

1 Tbs. soy sauce

1 package of tofu, cut into cubes

Directions

Make couscous with chicken broth (instead of water; follow directions on box).

In wok, stir-fry garlic, ginger, scallions, zucchinis, and tomato, until softened.

Add soy sauce and tofu.

Heat through.

Serve on couscous.

Dear Our Lady of Weight Loss,

I can't even say the "E" word, much less do it! It stems back to my childhood. I got a doctor's note each and every year excusing me from gym. And I keep hearing that I absolutely must move. I don't want to, but I guess I have to. Where should I begin? ~Motionless in Milwaukee

Dear Motionless,

You're going to have to make a pretty big mental shift here that may be even harder than the actual exercise program that you are going to slowly, happily, and successfully swing into. Make it a fun exploration. Sample a bunch of different exercise options. Try yoga one week, Pilates the next, walking, rock climbing, bicycling, weight lifting, boxing, and so on. The choices are endless. Bottom line: If you don't move, stretch, and exercise, you're going to be faced with a body that sags, drags, and lags. ~Our Lady of Weight Loss

Kick No. 31

Our Lady of Extreme Happiness

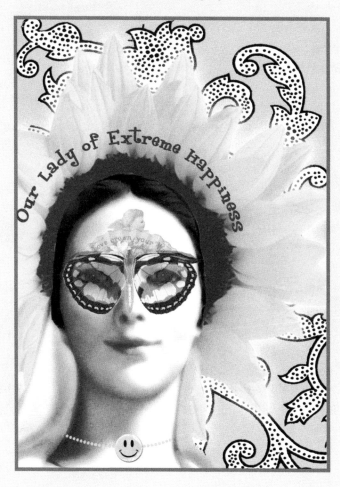

"Happiness always looks small while you hold it in your hands, but let it go, and you learn at once how big and precious it is."

~Maxim Gorky

MOTIVATIONAL MUSING
Foods That Make Us Happy

What is happiness? Are we as happy as we make up our minds to be? Is there truly an opportunity to find something positive in every event and everyone? I'd like to believe that to be true, although, I confess, some situations are more of a challenge than others.

It seems that happiness is, to a large degree, a choice—a state of mind. Attitude is enormously important. It is not our circumstances that make us unhappy; rather, it is our thoughts that cause us to be unhappy.

Yet happiness is also connected to two key mood regulators that our brain produces—serotonin and noradrenaline.

Serotonin is a mood enhancer that has an effect on pain, pleasure, anxiety, panic, arousal, and sleep patterns. Noradrenaline is a chemical that elevates our moods and affects aggression, stress, and anxiety. The more concentrated the amounts of these two chemicals, the happier we feel.

How does food enter the picture? Recent research has confirmed that there is a link between eating certain foods and feeling better, relaxed, and yes, even happy! What are these foods? Some proteins, yes—but carbohydrates, as well!

Carbohydrates carry a key amino acid, tryptophan, to our brains. Once there, tryptophan does its thing, and both noradrenaline and serotonin are produced. Our moods are given a bit of a boost.

Feeling blue? Here's a couple of fun foods that will give you a lift!

- Bananas. Bananas are loaded with magnesium, which reduces anxiety and helps you to sleep better.

- Oranges. Two glasses of freshly squeezed orange juice can help to lessen nervousness and bad moods. Lack of vitamin C, which affects noradrenaline levels, can make you crabby and low.

- Brazilian Walnuts. Brazilian walnuts are rich in selenium, which is related to a pleasant disposition. You need to eat only one or two walnuts to feel their effects. Wow! They're powerful!

- Chocolate. Ninety percent of women crave chocolate. Chocolate has a soothing effect. Just the taste alone brings pleasure. For weight-loss purposes, stick with dark chocolate in small and savored amounts.

- Turkey. This protein is a great source of tyrosine amino acid, which produces concentrated amounts of dopamine and nor-adrenaline.

- Water. Dehydration is a common cause for feeling tired, cranky, and depressed. When the body is dehydrated, the blood flow to the organs slows and functions decrease. That's scary! Don't just drink when you're thirsty. Approximately eight glasses per day is the suggested amount.

Tasty Tidbit Other than eating bananas, there are some things that you could do to increase your level of happiness.

Goals. What are your goals? What do you want to accomplish? Write out your lifetime goals and short-term goals. Goals give purpose and meaning to our lives.

Laugh. If you look for the funny side of life, you'll most likely find it.

Forgive and forget. It's difficult to feel happy if your heart is filled with bitterness, anger, or even hatred. Forgive yourselves first, and then the rest of the lot.

Give stuff away. Happiness is not about having more. Give of yourself.

Work on your relationships. We all need good relationships to share both the good and the bad times. A joy shared is a joy doubled. A problem shared is a problem halved.

Walk, run, skate. Exercise always makes us feel better. Get your endorphins pumping.

Faith. Lasting happiness cannot exist without faith. Faith creates peace of mind; it frees us from fear and anxiety. It leads us to deep places within.

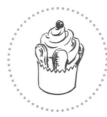

WEIGHTY CONFESSION

Forgive Me for I Have Sinned

I walked into the kitchen to get the step stool, but before I could remember what I was doing there, I made two pieces of cinnamon toast and gobbled them up.

All Is Forgiven.

Move On.

Blasphemous Banana Sundae

Ingredients

2 tsps. butter

2 tsps. sugar substitute

2 bananas

1 Tbs. rum extract

1 scoop of vanilla ice milk (light ice cream)

Directions

In a medium-size frying pan, melt butter and sugar substitute until blended. Don't burn it!

Cut the banana the long way and then in half (4 pieces) and sauté each side until light brown. Place banana pieces on plate. Add a few drops of rum extract to the sauce that remains in the frying pan. Mix it up and pour over the banana pieces. Place all on 1 scoop of vanilla ice cream—the light stuff (and one scoop only).

To die for!

Nutrition Facts

Serving Size (221g)
Servings Per Container 2

Amount Per Serving

Calories 310   Calories from Fat 100

	% Daily Value*
Total Fat 11g	**17%**
Saturated Fat 7g	**35%**
Trans Fat 0g	
Cholesterol 50mg	**17%**
Sodium 90mg	**4%**
Total Carbohydrate 50g	**17%**
Dietary Fiber 3g	**12%**
Sugars 35g	
Protein 5g	

Vitamin A 15%	•	Vitamin C 15%
Calcium 15%	•	Iron 4%

*Percent Daily Values are based on a 2,000 calorie diet. Your daily values may be higher or lower depending on your calorie needs:

	Calories	2,000	2,500
Total Fat	Less Than	65g	80g
Saturated Fat	Less Than	20g	25g
Cholesterol	Less Than	300mg	300 mg
Sodium	Less Than	2,400mg	2,400mg
Total Carbohydrate		300g	375g
Dietary Fiber		25g	30g

Calories per gram:
Fat 9 • Carbohydrate 4 • Protein 4

SACRED ASSIGNMENT

The Happiness Circle

Sit quietly, close your eyes, and just for a minute or two concentrate on the word *happiness*. When thoughts of happiness surface, open your eyes and either write the word *happiness* in the center of a piece of paper or use the template below. What comes to mind when you imagine that you feel happy? What are your associations to happiness? Write them in the happiness circle (or around the word happiness on your paper). Don't think; just go with your first thoughts about happiness.

Note: You might be surprised to see what does not enter the happiness picture. I've yet to find someone who equated happiness with gorging oneself!

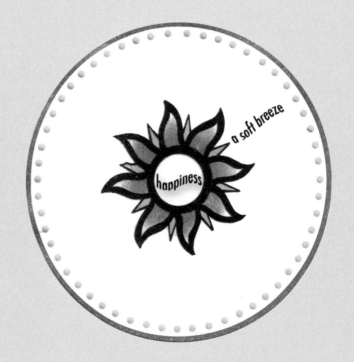

Kick No. 32

Our Lady of Dreamscapes and X-Files

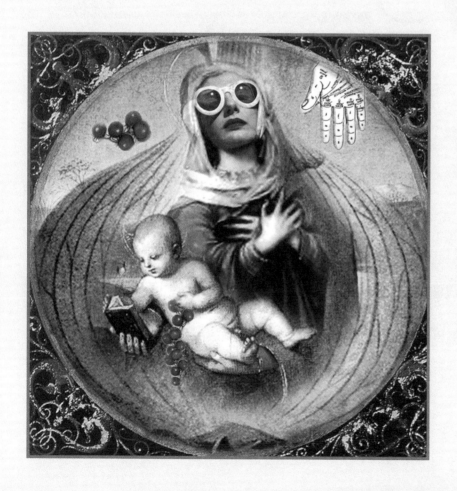

"Dreams are answers to questions we haven't yet figured out how to ask."

~X-Files

fa T oid

Five minutes after the
end of the dream, half
the content is forgotten.
After ten minutes,
90 percent is lost.

MOTIVATIONAL MUSING

To Dream the Impossible Dream

I dreamed that I woke up naturally thin.

In our dreams we can be anybody, go anywhere, do anything. We can defy science! We can eat as much pizza as we like and gain not even an ounce. Ahhh. To dream the impossible dream.

What are dreams?

Where do they come from?

And what do bananas symbolize?

According to Wikipedia, dreaming is the "subjective experience of imaginary images, sounds/voices, words, thoughts, or sensations during sleep, usually involuntarily. Dreams are a language of imagery. This imagery ranges from the normal to the surreal; in fact, dreams often provoke artistic and other forms of inspiration."

Dreams have been an area of study dating back to 4000 B.C. The Ancient Greeks and Freud thought that dreaming of food symbolized sexuality. Food represents what we take in. It often refers to the way we nourish our spirituality.

There are many distinct qualities about certain foods that can help us to determine their meaning in our dreams. For instance, popcorn suggests that we are full of ideas, eating pizza may epitomize idyllic times with family and friends, and bananas, yes, are thought to represent repressed sexual desires.

Here's a miniguide to some of the foods we dream about (to be ingested with a grain of salt).

- **Butter.** If you can see or taste butter in your dream, it implies that you are seeking gratification. Treat yourself to one of life's pleasures.
- **Candy.** Candy represents the special delicacies of life. It also symbolizes sensuality and forbidden pleasure.
- **Chocolate.** You may need to practice self-control. The presence of chocolate in your dream may mean that you are indulging in too many excesses.
- **Frozen foods.** Frozen foods may imply your emotions are cold and your ways are frigid! Brrrrrrr . . .
- **Ham.** Caution, curves ahead. Ham signifies that you are headed for some emotional difficulties.
- **Jelly.** To dream that you are eating jelly signifies pleasant surprises to come.
- **Omelet.** Omelets signify betrayal. Beware of those who flatter falsely!
- **Pickle.** The presence of a pickle may be representative of the penis. Sexual messages from the unconscious are bubbling to the surface.
- **Raspberry.** Raspberries foretell dangerous but interesting affairs ahead. Very intriguing!
- **Wine.** Wine signifies festivity, celebration, and companionship.

When analyzing your dreams, you should also consider your personal associations to foods. Some may stem from childhood memories. And then again, sometimes a piece of cake is just a piece of cake.

Beware: Food dreams can be triggered by dieting!

Nutrition Facts

Serving Size (454g)
Servings Per Container 4

Amount Per Serving

Calories 290	Calories from Fat 60

	% Daily Value*
Total Fat 6g	**9%**
Saturated Fat 0g	**0%**
Trans Fat 0g	
Cholesterol 0mg	**0%**
Sodium 780mg	**33%**
Total Carbohydrate 44g	**15%**
Dietary Fiber 13g	**52%**
Sugars 9g	
Protein 14g	

Vitamin A 30%	•	Vitamin C 140%	
Calcium 10%	•	Iron 30%	

*Percent Daily Values are based on a 2,000 calorie diet. Your daily values may be higher or lower depending on your calorie needs:

		Calories	2,000	2,500
Total Fat	Less Than		65g	80g
Saturated Fat	Less Than		20g	25g
Cholesterol	Less Than		300mg	300 mg
Sodium	Less Than		2,400mg	2,400mg
Total Carbohydrate			300g	375g
Dietary Fiber			25g	30g

Calories per gram:
Fat 9 • Carbohydrate 4 • Protein 4

RIGHTEOUS RECIPE

Iron Mike's Macho Two-Bean Mix-Up

Ingredients

6–8 tomatoes, diced

juice of 2–3 limes

1 medium red onion, diced

1–2 cups canned chickpeas, drained

1–2 cups canned black beans, drained

1 Tbs. olive oil

kosher salt (to taste)

fresh ground black pepper (to taste)

2–4 cloves garlic, minced (to taste)

green pepper, diced (optional)

red pepper, diced (optional)

1–2 green onions, sliced thin (optional)

This is really easy and delicious. Just dice, drain, squeeze, and mince, then shake all ingredients as instructed above—together. Let marinate for at least 1 hour (if you can stand it), and then enjoy. ~Iron Mike

Dear Our Lady of Weight Loss,

I had a dream last night. My friend and I were standing next to the refrigerator in my kitchen. The door mysteriously swung open, and inside, sitting on the top shelf—all in a row—sat three beautiful lemons. My friend said, "They look juicy and delicious." We each took one, but on closer examination they were soft and a bit moldy—and lemons aren't something I would just bite into. Nevertheless, foodie that I am, I could not resist. I peeled off some of the skin and took a bite. Yikes—it was rotten. I spit it out and woke up. What do you make of that?!
~Bitter Lemon

Dear Bitter Lemon,

Food in dreams often symbolizes emotional nourishment. Although I am not a licensed, certified dream therapist, here's what I think. I am wondering what or who your friend might represent. Dreams are not always about the actual person or object or event that you are dreaming. The lemons in a row may well symbolize order. Does your life look like it's in order, but at closer examination are you having a difficult time, perhaps in communicating with someone? Has a sour taste been left in your mouth by a friend or relative or situation? Having said that, next time you see your friend, should she offer you a lemon, I'd definitely pass!
~Our Lady of Weight Loss

Our Lady of Colorful Appetites

"Guys would
sleep with a
bicycle if it had
the right color
lip gloss on."

~Tori Amos

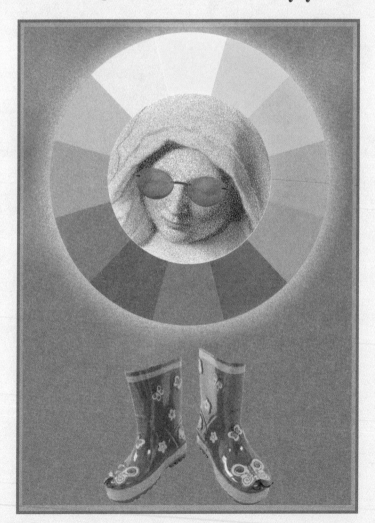

196

faToid

The human eye
is capable of
differentiating ten
million colors.

MOTIVATIONAL MUSING
Color and Our Appetites!

Color adds excitement and emotion to our lives. Everything from the clothes we wear (you mean there's more than black?) to the pictures we paint to our moods and, yes, even to our appetites revolve around and are affected by color.

What Is Color?

Color is the by-product of light, as it is reflected or absorbed and experienced by the human eye and processed by the human brain.

Without light, there would be no color. Light is made up of energy waves. These waves are grouped together and are called the spectrum (the rainbow!). The wavelengths of light are not actually colored, but they create the sensation of color.

How Does Color Affect Our Appetites?

Orange is a stimulant. It stimulates emotions, thoughts, conversation, and appetite.

Red stimulates our appetites as well, and restaurants often incorporate both red and orange into their design plan. Red clothing may get us some attention, but it also makes us look heavier!

Green, the strongest and the most universal color in nature, signifies hope, life, youth, and renewal, and it is the easiest on the eyes. It has been known to improve vision.

Blue foods are rare (blueberries come to mind; anything else?). When our ancestors were out foraging, they found that the toxic or spoiled foods were most often blue, black, or purple. Therefore, the color blue is a natural appetite suppressant! And—for whatever reason—studies show that weight lifters find handling heavier weights easier in blue gyms.

While **yellow** is considered an optimistic color, it seems to be the color of rooms in which people most often lose their tempers and babies cry! If overused, it can be overpowering and hard on the eyes. Nevertheless, yellow enhances concentration, and—it accelerates metabolism.

And, finally—**black.** We all know that black clothing absolutely makes us look slimmer!

WEIGHTY CONFESSION

Forgive Me for I Have Sinned

It was my intention to play tennis at my in-laws' country club, but alas, I lay by the pool like a lox—all day long. My only activity was slathering on the SPF 45 suntan lotion and getting up to serve myself at the ice cream sundae buffet—twice! Hot fudge, candy chips, whip cream, the works. Dee-liciousssss.

All Is Forgiven.
Move On.

Pious Project
THE BATTLE OF THE BULGE

You bet. It is a battle. And sometimes you've got to gear up and arm yourself. This helmet protects us from the evil-fat-doers and reminds us that we're gonna' win.

SUPPLIES

1 army helmet liner (you can find it at an Army-Navy store—it looks like a helmet but it's actually the liner. The helmet weighs a ton.)

white gesso
sponge brush
red paint
small number 1 paintbrush
toy soldiers
stencil
pencil
black paint
craft cement glue

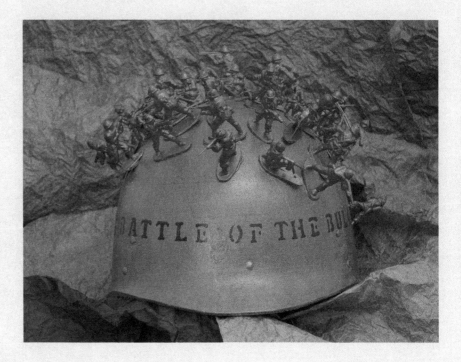

INSTRUCTIONS

Paint the helmet with a layer of gesso (it's a primer) with sponge brush.

When it dries, paint a layer of red (with the sponge brush; you can wash out the white or use another one).

While the helmet is drying, you can use the number 1 brush and paint the soldiers the same red.

With stencil and pencil, write out "The Battle of the Bulge."

Fill in with black paint using your number 1 paintbrush.

When dry, place some craft cement on the bottom of the soldiers and glue them to the helmet in a random fashion. You'll have to hold them in place until they dry, especially the ones that are walking down the sides.

In the end, the soldiers can defy gravity (with the help of a little cement glue).

You can defy sweets (with the help of Our Lady)!

Our Lady of the Long Hot Soak

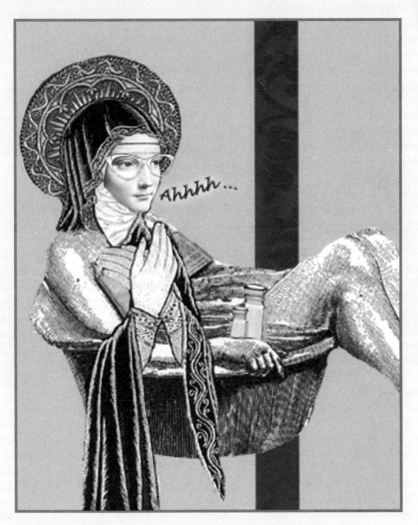

"Everything is a miracle. It is a miracle that one does not dissolve in one's bath like a lump of sugar."

~Pablo Picasso

MOTIVATIONAL MUSING
The Long Hot Soak

Bathing is an ancient custom.

We know that the Romans, Babylonians, and Egyptians practiced bathing, but no one knows who enjoyed the first hot soak or when. Some say that humans learned of the healing nature of the hot bath when they found animals sitting in natural hot springs healing (and licking) their wounds.

A long, hot soak provides a space in which to relax, promotes health by stimulating circulation, and literally cleanses the body. Baths help to restore our mental and spiritual well-being.

And the bath is a natural no-food zone. It is quite possibly the only room in the house that I do not think to bring food into nor do I ruminate on the topic! Truly, who can negotiate a burger and fries while soaking?

The bath presents a perfect opportunity do so some deep breathing exercises, get in touch with your body, and immerse yourself in thin thoughts.

As your breathing becomes slower and deeper and the heat penetrates your body, visualize your fat melting away.

How to Set the Stage

Turn off the phone.

Turn on some inspiring meditative music.

Light a forest of fragrant candles.

Add essential oils of your choice—and/or . . .

Fragrant bubbles. (Best to use natural bubble bath products versus the mainstream kind that may share some of the ingredients of laundry detergent!)

Run bath water that is a bit warmer than your body temperature.

Tasty Tidbit **Some things to think about when deciding on bath scents:**

Lavender at night promotes sleep.

Rosemary helps circulation and warms the body.

Citrus stimulates the body.

Eucalyptus relieves muscle aches and pains.

Patchouli and sage are great for relaxation.

Dear Our Lady of Weight Loss,

My husband works nights and usually arrives home at 5:00 A.M. When he arrived home this morning, he woke me up to show me that he'd picked up a half gallon of my favorite Rocky Road ice cream. I couldn't resist. I got up and joined him at the kitchen table. We polished off the entire container. Weight loss is a challenge for me and this was a major setback. I feel awful. I never should have gotten up. I am weak and have no willpower. I'm hoping you can encourage me to get back on the wagon. ~On the Rocky Road to Weight Loss

Dear Rocky Road,

I think you're blaming the victim here. And that victim would be you. Your husband set you up. It was sabotage and a totally unsupportive act on his behalf. Why did he bring it into the house? I've said it before, and I'll say it again. There is no such thing as willpower; it's want power. You have to want to lose weight enough not to have Rocky Road ice cream in the house. Sometimes when people lose weight, their partners are threatened by the change. Perhaps you could sit down and have a talk. Ask him politely not to bring home goodies. My guess is that he doesn't need it either! ~Our Lady of Weight Loss

RIGHTEOUS RECIPE
Bath Salts

NOT FOR CONSUMPTION

*G*ive yourself an inexpensive vacation.

Mix 1 cup of Epsom salts with 1 cup of baking soda.

Add two tablespoons of liquid glycerin (which can be purchased at a craft store, soap store, or on-line) and a couple of drops of your favorite essential oil.

Light a couple of candles; put on some "light" music, add your bath salt mix to your hot water, and relax. Ahhhhh . . . Let it all go.

Kick No. 35

Our Lady Is Made of Heavenly Spice

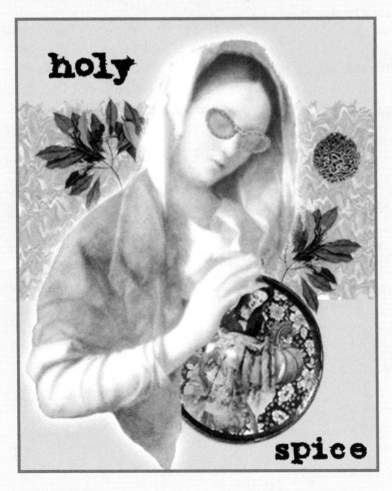

"Wish I had time for just one more bowl of chili."
~Alleged dying words of Kit Carson

MOTIVATIONAL MUSING
Spice It Up, Cowboy

Sound the five-alarm chili bells and whistles. Spicy foods can aid your weight-loss efforts!

According to a study published in the *British Journal of Nutrition*, capsaicin, a compound found in red peppers that makes them red hot, causes people to eat less.

Thirteen women who ate a breakfast spiced up with red peppers ate less than they normally would at breakfast and throughout the day. Ten men who ate spiced up snacks before lunch consumed less calories during lunch and throughout the rest of their day. Hot red peppers act as an appetite suppressant and increase the number of calories burned.

Further, a study from the 1980s found that eating just one spiced up, red-hot meal can boost your metabolism by up to 25 percent. And this burnin' spike can last for up to three hours!

It's the capsaicin that is found in jalapeño and cayenne peppers that temporarily stimulates your body to release more stress hormones (i.e., adrenaline), speeding up your metabolism and causing those calories to burn!

What to do? Spice it up, baby. It's likely that the spiciness of the food makes us feel full. Double benefit. We're burning more calories and eating less.

And triple benefit: It's been my experience that the more burnin' hot it is, the more water needed to put out that five-alarm blaze. For those who find drinking water a challenge, here's a way to work it in and get it down the hatch!

Tasty Tidbit How to make your day red-hot:

Sprinkle hot peppers in your soup.

Layer hot peppers in your sandwiches.

Add jalapeño to your favorite recipes.

Dear Our Lady of Weight Loss,

I am able to say "no, thank you" to fattening foods, but over and over again, I have real problems not eating too much of the healthy, low-fat, low-cal stuff. If a portion of something is under 250 calories, I'm more than likely going to load up my plate at least three times; whereas, if something was 750 calories, I'd never even go near it. Any suggestions? ~Low-Cal Overeater

Dear Low-Cal Overeater,

It's really great that you know where your challenges lie. And you must want to do something about it, or you wouldn't have written to me. So, here's my suggestion. If you just can't help yourself, and it's too much for you (and you're not alone) to have the entire bowl of food on the table, then serve your one portion and freeze the rest before you sit down and eat. Out of sight, out of mind. Buy as many items as you can that are preportioned. If you cook, package them yourself in portion sizes. ~Our Lady of Weight Loss

Pious Projects
NON-PIGGY BANK

I must have said and continue to say "No, thank you" to offers of food about eight zillion times a day. *No! I am not exaggerating.* You'd think the scales of injustice would be appreciative of my efforts and automatically reward me. Yet, if I cave—even just once—to the sweet temptation of a hot fudge sundae, all my righteous efforts are sugared and fattened away.

I wanted a reward! So, I made a non-piggy bank and paid myself one dollar for each and every non-piggy no thank you I uttered. When my non-piggy is filled with cash, I count it joyfully and either go for a manicure or buy lipstick.

My non-piggy bank changed the focus of my no-thank-yous from deprivation to fun! I started looking for people to offer me things.

"Aren't you going to offer me some of that key lime pie?" I asked a friend, who I'd irrationally labeled a food pusher the week before. She looked at me quizzically and apprehensively inquired, "Would you like a slice of pie?"

"Non merci, je suis à la diète," I cheerfully answered in French, adding another level of flavor to my no-thank-you. I kept count of my no-thank-yous, and when I got home that night, I had twenty extra no-thank-you bucks to add to my jar!! (I borrowed the money from my husband.)

How to make a non-piggy bank:

SUPPLIES

1 glass jar (Mine was once jam-packed with sweet gherkins pickles. Sweet gherkin pickles are only 15 calories each, if you are just dying for a quick mix of sweet, sour, and crunchy! And they are a treat that I have no trouble controlling. One or two sweet gherkins do it for me.)

1 inspirational picture

opaque paint markers (These pens are filled with colorful paints, and there's no fuss or muss.)

INSTRUCTIONS

Clean the jar. Remove the label. And paint away.

As you can see, I first pasted my favorite Our Lady on the jar. She guides and inspires—*always!* And then I painted the words "*Non merci, je suis à la diète,*" followed by some decorative touches.

You can go wild. Make swirls. Dots. Triangles.

You can use stickers as well. Stamps. Anything!

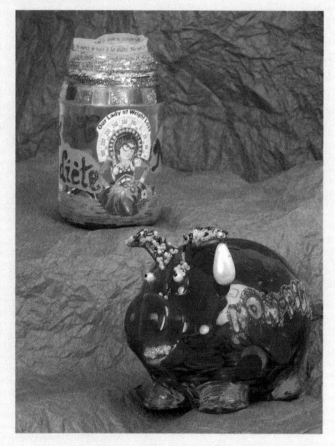

Our Lady Is Stressed Out!

"There cannot be
a stressful crisis
next week.
My schedule is
already full."
~Henry Kissinger

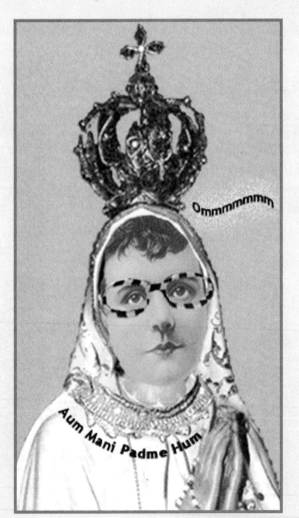

MOTIVATIONAL MUSING
Stressed to My Last Nerve

faToid

Worry and stress affect the circulation, the heart, the glands, the whole nervous system, and profoundly affect heart action.

are you stressed? Irritable? Having trouble sleeping? Do you feel like screaming? Crying? Pouring a jug of water over your boss's head?

We all feel stressed from time to time, so it's essential to have an arsenal of coping mechanisms at hand. Instead of heading for the refrigerator, here are some stress management tips that should help ease the pressures of life!

- **Breathe.** No kidding; take in a few deep cleansing breaths and slow down.
- **Change your routine.** If you've been sitting all day thinking, get up and get physical. Take a walk, stretch. And if you've been lifting heavy boxes from sunrise to sunset, sit down and think deep thoughts.
- **Keep things in perspective.** When you're in a twist about something, ask yourself, "Will this matter in ten years? Five years? Tomorrow?" Most of what frazzles us is just passing through. Wave good-bye to it.
- **Smile and laugh a lot.** Every chance you get.
- **Prioritize.** Concentrate on one task at a time. Multitasking can be nerve-racking.
- **Don't put off what can be done today.** Get those unpleasant tasks out of the way as soon as possible, lest they hang over your head.

- ➤ **Call a friend**. Talk it through. Vent. (I use the Five People Plan. When stressed or upset, I tell five people about it. By the time I get to the fifth person, I'm so over it and really tired of hearing myself!)
- ➤ **Add vitamin C to your diet**. Studies show that vitamin C knocks out the secretion of stress hormones.
- ➤ **Do something creative!** Relieve some tension by using your imagination. Garden, read, sing, dance, paint, draw, play an instrument, make macaroni art—anything you can think of that takes you away from the stress and opens your mind to the possibilities.
- ➤ **Chant**. "Aum Mani Padme Hum" (pronounced "Om mahnay pahdmay hoom"). The most popular translation is "Hail the jewel in the lotus." It is recited by Tibetan Buddhists to invoke Chenrezi, the Bodhisattva of Compassion.

Tasty Tidbit **Our Lady of Weight Loss's List of Top Ten Stressors**

1. A scale that says that I weigh more than I think I do!!! Seriously, it must be broken.
2. Water retention.
3. Bad hair day. (Does frizzy hair weigh more?)
4. Dinner at a friend's home who says she'll cook light but doesn't. (Saboteur!)
5. Chipped nails the day of my manicure.
6. Chocolate gifts. (What are they thinking?)
7. Being hungry.
8. Tight pants and/or busted zipper.
9. Holiday meals with the family. Love 'em, though. I do.
10. People talking on cell phones in restaurants. (It makes me want to drown out the noise with bread.)

WEIGHTY CONFESSION
Forgive Me for I Have Sinned

I was making dinner for friends, and I just couldn't stop myself from tasting it every two seconds, so I took the masking tape from the closet and taped my mouth shut! It wouldn't have been so bad had my husband and children arrived home earlier than expected, and for an instant they became terrified that I'd been mugged!

All Is Forgiven.
Move On.

Pious Project
THE STRESSLESS GARDEN

It's Thin Thyme! Grow Your Own

I've been working on my indoor herb garden.

I started with thyme because it was what was available to me at the local market for under two dollars. It was a tiny, little stalk with a few green leaves. I brought it home, watered it, talked to it, and repotted it in a special terra-cotta planter. Special, indeed! I decoupaged thin messages all over it—from "Thin Thyme" to "Bite out of Life" to "Knockout."

My thin thyme loves her new home. Her leaves gracefully cascade onto the table, and her thyme smell is divine. I can pinch a bit here and there for Our Lady–approved soups and stews! And every time I look at her (which is often), she reminds me that it's thin thyme!!

SUPPLIES

1 1" sponge brush
heavy gel (gloss) medium (acts as glue and glossy finish)
newspaper (foreign language with color is always fun or black and
    white, your choice)
1 terra-cotta planter with one terra-cotta base
1 magazine
1 tube bronze acrylic paint
1 herb plant with potting soil

INSTRUCTIONS

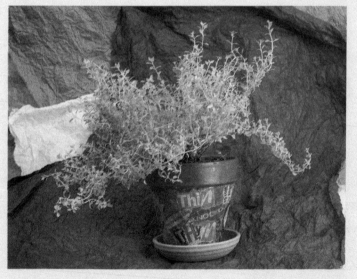

Using sponge brush, brush on layer of heavy gel medium.

Rip newspaper into small pieces ($\frac{1}{2}$" to 1") and paste onto terra-cotta planter. (You're creating a haphazard bottom layer of graphics.)

Rip through your magazine, looking for meaningful words and/or phrases. Tear them out and paste on top of newspaper.

If you want to add a "glaze," mix a little bronze acrylic paint with some heavy gel medium and paint over words.

Plant your herbs.

Water them, talk sweetly to them, and watch them grow!

Kick No. 37

Our Lady of Complete and Utter Silence

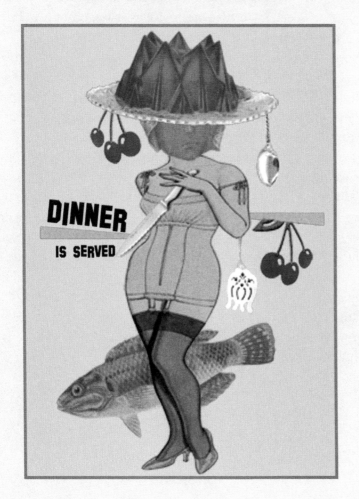

"Let us be silent,
that we may
hear the whispers
of the gods."
~Ralph Waldo
Emerson

faToid

There are nine thousand
taste buds on the human
tongue.

MOTIVATIONAL MUSING
The Silent Dinner

Ready to expand your horizons and enter the Land of Silence? Silent, meditative meals give us an opportunity to be present, experience our food mindfully, and reflect.

When we eat without speaking, we are free to experience the uniqueness of each bite and perhaps to consider the many elements that made our meal possible—the sun, rain, soil, air, and even the people who may have come into contact with it in one way or another.

We can appreciate the texture, flavor, aroma, and look of the food, and focus on how each morsel affects our bodies. We are able to experience the rhythm in which we are eating and the physical sensation as the food passes through our lips, how it feels on our tongues, sliding down our throats, and even how the food feels breaking down in our stomachs.

Through silent eating, we will not only be more aware of the moment, mindful of what we are doing, but we are also able to slow our eating and, in turn, eat less.

If ingesting an entire meal in silence is too overwhelming a concept for you, start with a piece of fruit, and if a whole piece of fruit is too much, how about one peanut?

Tasty Tidbit **How to Make the Most of a Silent Meal**

Be present. With awareness, wakefulness, silently say grace.

A simple start. Take the food of your choice, something healthful, please. Spend a few moments just looking at it and appreciating its origins, its color, its texture and smell.

A gentle roll. Gently roll it around in your mouth, feel it with your tongue. Notice how your salivary glands have come to action.

Contemplate. Appreciate the interconnectedness of the earth, the soil, the rain, the food, and yourself.

Bring it on (slowly). Move to the next course, the appetizer (and so forth). Stay present with each and every bite.

Share the experience. If you are eating in silence with friends or family, ring a soft bell signifying the end of the silent meal. Silently say a prayer of gratitude. And then . . . let the chatting begin.

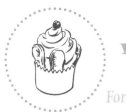

WEIGHTY CONFESSION

Forgive Me for I Have Sinned

In a desperate moment, I took teething crackers out of my toddler's chubby hands and popped them into my mouth. I told him I would give him money instead.

All Is Forgiven.
Move On.

Pious Project

THROW A SILENT DINNER PARTY

I had my reservations about inviting my friends over and hosting a silent dinner. Not only am I regular chatty Cathy, but my friends and family are motor-mouth Mabels, each and every one! They like to talk as much as I do. In the end, it was a lot of fun. When the timer went off, and it was time to talk again, no one wanted to be the first to break the silence. What a hoot. It went on for another seven minutes (I counted!).

A word to the wise. Remember, silent dinners are supposed to be free of all noise. If at all possible do not invite any heavy-duty schlurpers. Oh, and assign jobs before the dinner begins. For example, you might want help clearing the table between courses. I made place cards with names and jobs on the backs of them. This way there'd be no confusion when it was time to clear the salad plates.

Menu: soup, salad, main course, dessert

To the left is a copy of my menu.

---

no schlurping * no laughing * no snorting * no talking * no loud open-mouthed chewing or humming * no lipsmacking * no snoring * no funny faces * no joking * no chuckling * no spitting * no choking *

OUR LADY OF WEIGHT LOSS'S SILENT DINNER PARTY

MENU

watermelon martinis

deviled eggs

love thyself pie

waldorf salad à la Our Lady

blasphemous banana sundae

And here's a copy of the invite. I sewed buttons onto the RSVP cards, and you can do the same for fun. The buttons will make their way back to you, and you can recycle them once again.

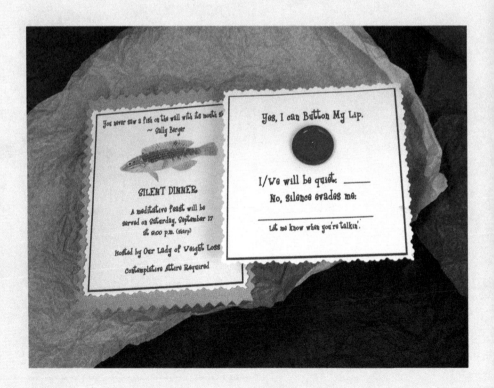

The invitation reads:

You never saw a fish on the wall with its mouth sh...
~ Sally Berger

SILENT DINNER

A meditative Feast will be
served on Saturday, September 17
at 9:00 p.m. (sharp)

Hosted by Our Lady of Weight Loss

Contemplative Attire Required

Yes, I can Button My Lip.

I/We will be quiet: _____
No, silence evades me: _____
_____
Let me know when you're talkin'.

Our Lady of Aromatherapy

"Smell is a
potent wizard
that transports
you across
thousands of
miles and all
the years you
have lived."
~Helen Keller

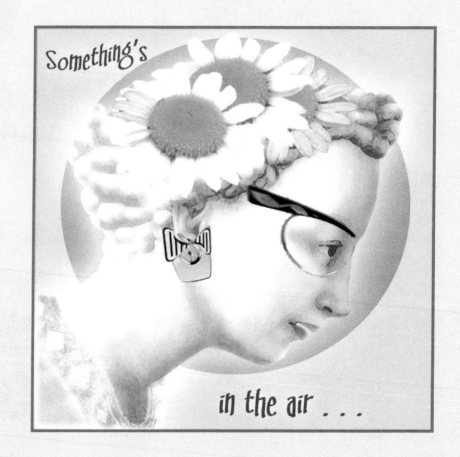

Something's In the Air

*A*romatherapy may not miraculously melt away the pounds, but there are heaps of evidence that aroma affects mood. And we all know how mood affects our eating!

What Is Aromatherapy?

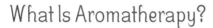

Aromatherapy means "treatment through senses." It is based on the ancient ritual of using essential oils to heal by therapeutically stimulating the nasal/olfactory senses through fragrance.

Aromatherapy can fight stress, soothe the mind, and lighten your mood. The association between smell and emotion are closely linked, and breathing in pleasurable scents can elicit positive responses in the brain, resulting in a sense of well-being.

Aromatherapy can also lessen our food cravings! A recent study at St. George's Hospital in London showed that vanilla might aid in weight loss. Overweight people who wore vanilla-scented skin patches reported that they ingested fewer sweets. Catherine Collins, a state registered dietician, concluded that strongly scented sweet vanilla candles or essence may have a similar effect. My home smells like a vanilla factory!

And—by massaging the appropriate essential oils into the skin—aromatherapy can ease aches and pains, heal burns, and even—some say—diminish cellulite! *(What? Did you say diminish cellulite?)*

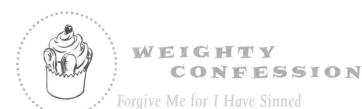

WEIGHTY CONFESSION

Forgive Me for I Have Sinned

Early last evening I sipped on a glass of cabernet sauvignon as I poured basmati rice into our fabulously expensive rice cooker. I added water and salt.

Just a bit of salt, I thought. But I was chitchatting (via telephone) with my dear friend Wendy (who has her last radiation treatment this morning). I must have put the salt in twice (maybe thrice?), because when it was done and I tasted it, the rice was beyond salty; beyond as salty as the time I sipped on soy sauce thinking it was ice tea. It was water-retention weight salty. Nevertheless, while still talking on the phone (for over an hour), I stood over the kitchen counter, sampling the rice one spoonful at a time until—lo 'n' behold—every one of those salty morsels was devoured.

I am puffy this morning, and I vow never to discuss heavy matters, on the phone or otherwise, while cooking or sampling food.

All Is Forgiven.
Move on.

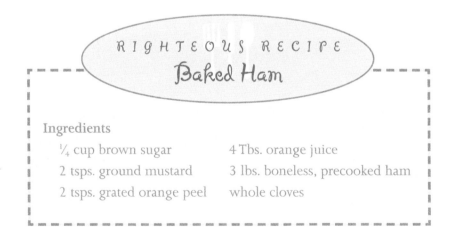

RIGHTEOUS RECIPE
Baked Ham

Ingredients

¼ cup brown sugar	4 Tbs. orange juice
2 tsps. ground mustard	3 lbs. boneless, precooked ham
2 tsps. grated orange peel	whole cloves

Nutrition Facts

Serving Size 3 oz. (94g)
Servings Per Container 16

Amount Per Serving

Calories 120	Calories from Fat 30

	% Daily Value*
Total Fat 3.5g	**5%**
Saturated Fat 1g	**5%**
Trans Fat 0g	
Cholesterol 35mg	**12%**
Sodium 920mg	**38%**
Total Carbohydrate 8g	**3%**
Dietary Fiber 0g	**0%**
Sugars 8g	
Protein 13g	

Vitamin A 0%	•	Vitamin C 30%
Calcium 0%	•	Iron 8%

*Percent Daily Values are based on a 2,000 calorie diet. Your daily values may be higher or lower depending on your calorie needs:

		Calories	2,000	2,500
Total Fat	Less Than		65g	80g
Saturated Fat	Less Than		20g	25g
Cholesterol	Less Than		300mg	300 mg
Sodium	Less Than		2,400mg	2,400mg
Total Carbohydrate			300g	375g
Dietary Fiber			25g	30g

Calories per gram:
Fat 9 • Carbohydrate 4 • Protein 4

Yes, there's sugar in the recipe, but one teaspoon of sugar is only 16 calories. That's one teaspoon, not one tablespoon! Once again, it's all about moderation. So if you don't go crazy and drink a cup of the gravy, you'll be all right.

Directions

Combine brown sugar, mustard, orange peel, and orange juice with a quick whisk.

Score top of ham. Stud with whole cloves.

Bake in 350° oven for 1 hour; baste with sugar mixture for the last 30 minutes.

Let stand 15 minutes and slice.

Kick No. 39

Our Lady Is Stronger Than Dirt

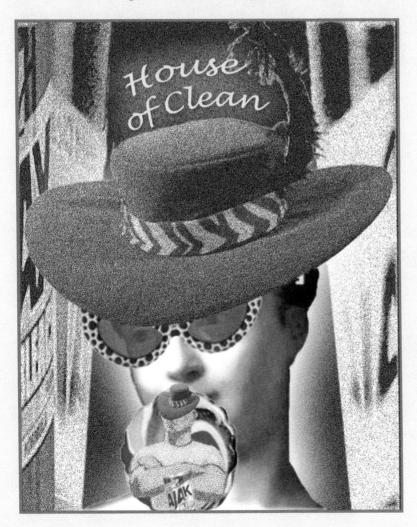

"I hate
housework!
You make the
beds, you do the
dishes—and six
months later you
have to start all
over again."
~ Joan Rivers

MOTIVATIONAL MUSING
Housework as Exercise!

Wanna polish off that piece of cake? Try polishing the dressers instead.

Given the amount of running around we all do, we barely have enough time to sleep, much less exercise and/or clean. But there is a great way to help squeeze thirty minutes of exercise into your day.

As the Mayo Clinic suggests, you can combine housework and exercise. They say, "Make household chores count. Mop the floor, scrub the bathtub or do other housework. The stretching and lifting are good exercise. Work at a fast pace to get your heart pumping."

Our Lady suggests we add one mammoth helping of music to the Mayo's housework as exercise workout program. As we know (see Exercise Tips for Exercise Flunkies, page 179), music activates the same feels good center of the brain that food does. If we could dust, mop, stretch, and sweat to the beat of Motown, we'd burn calories, have a clean house, and get those morphinelike substances that our body produces that enhance the immune system, relieve pain, reduce stress, and postpone the aging process pumping too.

What songs does Our Lady squat, bend, push, pull, and lift to? Aretha Franklin's "Respect" and "Pink Cadillac," Gwen Stefani's "Rich Girl," OutKast's "The Love Below," and Tina Turner's "Proud Mary."

Tasty Tidbit **Housework as exercise is not a new concept. In October 1901, *Good Housekeeping* published an article entitled "Housework as Exercise." The author was an unnamed teacher of physical culture. Her message was for us to "unbutton those tight collars, take off the corsets and petticoats, hike up those long skirts and pull the blinds. Whenever possible wear a gymnasium suit for scrubbing and sweeping."**

Housework as Exercise Calorie Chart

Activity	Calories burned per hour
cooking	80
(No tasting while cooking!)	
ironing	60
mopping floors	110
rearranging furniture	200
scrubbing floors	200
vacuuming	85
washing dishes (by hand)	60
washing windows	150

WEIGHTY CONFESSION

Forgive Me for I Have Sinned

My husband recently found a pillowcase laced with chocolate stains. I said nothing. When he asked if I had taken any chocolate to bed, I said nothing. I simply shook my head from side to side, as I squirreled my chocolate Fruit 'n' Nut bar under my head.
~Lindsey

All Is Forgiven.
Move On.

Nutrition Facts

Serving Size (273g)
Servings Per Container 8

Amount Per Serving

Calories 310   Calories from Fat 25

	% Daily Value*
Total Fat 3g	**5%**
Saturated Fat 0g	**0%**
Trans Fat 0g	
Cholesterol 0mg	**0%**
Sodium 380mg	**16%**
Total Carbohydrate 61g	**20%**
Dietary Fiber 7g	**28%**
Sugars 9g	
Protein 13g	

Vitamin A 20%	•	Vitamin C 100%
Calcium 4%	•	Iron 20%

*Percent Daily Values are based on a 2,000 calorie diet. Your daily values may be higher or lower depending on your calorie needs:

		Calories	2,000	2,500
Total Fat	Less Than		65g	80g
Saturated Fat	Less Than		20g	25g
Cholesterol	Less Than		300mg	300 mg
Sodium	Less Than		2,400mg	2,400mg
Total Carbohydrate			300g	375g
Dietary Fiber			25g	30g

Calories per gram:
Fat 9 • Carbohydrate 4 • Protein 4

RIGHTEOUS RECIPE
Linguine à la Garbanzo

Ingredients

3 garlic cloves, minced

3 medium zucchinis, sliced

1 large red pepper, sliced

1 large onion, diced

2 tsp. olive oil

1 28-oz. can crushed tomatoes (Italian herb seasoning)

1 15.5-oz. can garbanzo beans, drained

16 oz. spinach linguine

Parmesan cheese (optional)

a handful of fresh Italian parsley.

Directions

In a large pot over medium heat, cook garlic, zucchini, red pepper, and onion in olive oil until tender, 10 minutes or so.

Add tomatoes and garbanzo beans.

Heat to boiling. Reduce heat to low; cover and simmer 30 minutes. Meanwhile, cook pasta as label directs.

Drain. Add sauce and serve with grated cheese, if desired.

Garnish with fresh Italian parsley.

Kick No. 40

Our Lady of the Waning Moon

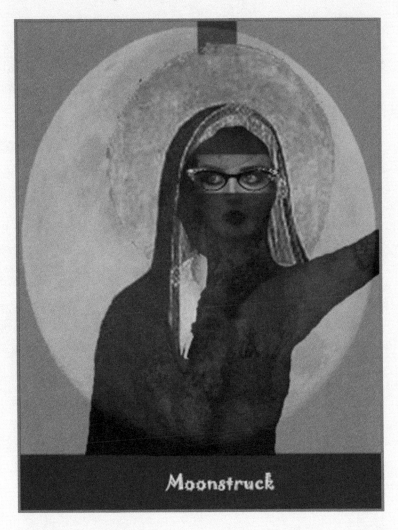

Moonstruck

"Seen from the moon we are all the same size."
~Multatuli (Eduard Douwers Dekker)

faⓉoid

A blue moon takes place
when the moon appears
twice within the same
calendar month. The
blue moon is considered
a "goal moon," at which
time you set specific
goals for yourself.

MOTIVATIONAL MUSING
Moonstruck

From prehistoric times through the present, the moon has held our imagination. The moon was our first timekeeper. The moon causes the ebb and flow of the tides; and because our bodies are 75 percent water, the moon also affects our emotions, moods, sleep patterns, and for women, our menstrual cycles.

The moon's cycle lasts twenty-eight days, and through those twenty-eight days the moon appears to transform itself from the tiny sliver of a new moon into the glistening luminosity of the full moon fourteen days later, and then slowly back into the dark moon.

The new moon (the waxing moon) is a time associated with beginnings and growth. If you want to bring new things into your life, to start a new project, to start anew—to bring a fresh start to your healthy food program, for example—the new moon phase presents a strong foundation on which to begin.

The full moon (the waning moon) presents a time of power. It is an excellent time to become aware of your negative thoughts. It is a time to overcome obstacles, to relinquish bad habits. It is a time of clearing.

New Moon/Full Moon Ritual

This is a fun exercise that can bring awareness and intention to your life.

There are two ways to perform this ritual: the simple way, and the deluxe version. The results will be the same. It's all a matter of finding what works best for you.

The key to this exercise is this: A pen together with paper can prove a powerful life tool.

If you choose the simple way, you will simply need a pen and paper.

However, if you choose the full deluxe ritual, you will need the following:

maroon-, red-, wine-, or orange-colored paper

white, orange, maroon, red, or wine pen or marker

1 dark red– or wine-colored candle

1 orange-colored candle

matches or a lighter

a glass candle holder that holds both candles comfortably

incense (your favorite scent)

a gemstone, such as carnelian or garnet (anything red)

wet fingers/candlesnuffer

The simple way. On the day of the new moon (any time that works for you) make a list of all the new things that you want to bring into your life. There is no right or wrong way to do this. My new moon list has covered everything from new glasses to a new home to a new point of view.

The deluxe version. Same as above, but you'll need to use the right color pen (listed above in your supply list) and paper, along with candles, etc. Again, you should write out a list of all the things you want to bring into your life. After you complete your list, pick three that resonate deeply. And then place your list under the plate that holds the candles, and with gemstone in hand, while candles and incense are burning, ask the universe for your three wishes.

> "I ask the universe to bring hot, steamy, love into my life."
>
> "I ask the universe to bring large sums of cash into my life."
>
> "I ask the universe to bring a new gourmet deli to my block that stocks light bread."

These are examples, of course, and you should create your own list. And be specific!

Repeat the wishes out loud three times. Let the candles burn for as long as you are focused on your wishes. Do not blow them out. Either wet your fingers and pinch the flame out, or use a snuffer.

Keep your ritual kit in a safe place. Save your list, and when you write next month's new moon list, be sure to compare. You may find that your priorities have shifted or that some of your list has manifested.

Fourteen days later, you can complete your full moon list. The full moon ritual is basically the same, except this time you want to make a list of everything you want out of your life. Again, there is no right or wrong way to do this. My list has ranged from ridding myself of bad hair days to overcoming illness.

Again, your requests should be as specific as possible and well thought out.

For example,

> "I ask the universe to rid me of bad hair days."

"They" say that 75 percent of what we write down happens. I'm not sure if it's pure magic or that when our desires come to light, our intention takes hold, and our actions change. Either way, change is a miraculous phenomenon that we are all capable of making happen.

New Moon Orzo with Spinach

Easy and yum delicious.

Ingredients

1 8-oz. box of orzo

1 lb. spinach

fresh garlic, diced, to taste

2 tsps. olive oil

1 red bell pepper, deseeded and chopped

salt and pepper, to taste

grated Parmesan cheese, to taste

Instructions:

Cook orzo al dente.

Sauté spinach and garlic in olive oil.

Toss all ingredients together.

Nutrition Facts

Serving Size (108g)
Servings Per Container 4

Amount Per Serving

Calories 240 Calories from Fat 30

	% Daily Value*
Total Fat 3g	5%
Saturated Fat 0.5g	3%
Trans Fat 0g	
Cholesterol 0mg	0%
Sodium 0mg	0%
Total Carbohydrate 46g	15%
Dietary Fiber 3g	12%
Sugars 4g	
Protein 8g	

Vitamin A 20%	• Vitamin C 100%
Calcium 2%	• Iron 10%

*Percent Daily Values are based on a 2,000 calorie diet. Your daily values may be higher or lower depending on your calorie needs:

		Calories	2,000	2,500
Total Fat	Less Than		65g	80g
Saturated Fat	Less Than		20g	25g
Cholesterol	Less Than		300mg	300 mg
Sodium	Less Than		2,400mg	2,400mg
Total Carbohydrate			300g	375g
Dietary Fiber			25g	30g

Calories per gram:
Fat 9 • Carbohydrate 4 • Protein 4

Dear Our Lady of Weight Loss,

My diet mind is a little confused. I've gained almost fifteen pounds since Christmas and get this—I actually don't mind. This is wildly unusual for me. I'm always conflicted about diets (or as Richard Simmons says, "Live-it," because who wants to "die-it"?). Eat when you're hungry and stop when you're full. Eat small bits of everything you really like so you don't feel deprived and binge. Love and enjoy food, put food in a tiny place and fill up on life. I'm tired of trying to be thin. It's exhausting. ~Richard's Girl

Dear Richard's Girl,

You bet, trying to be thin is exhausting! How about truly getting into a healthy lifestyle? Plan one week of healthy living and see how it goes. Walk, breathe, enjoy, and I can tell you from my own experience, if you primarily eat low-fat, low-cal foods (fruits, vegetables, grains), and concentrate on feeling good, you'll be hard-pressed to gain weight. I promise you that being healthy is fun, exciting, and gratifying. ~Our Lady of Weight Loss

Kick No. 41

Our Lady of the Office Manifesto

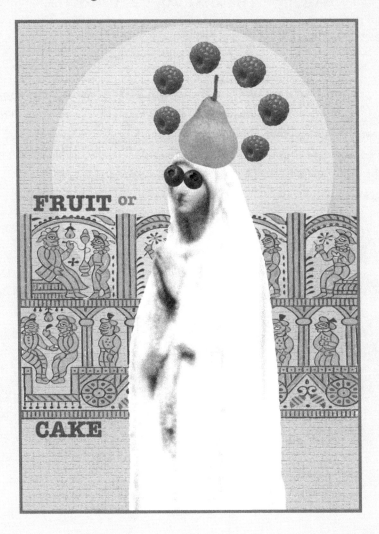

"Eating's going to
be a whole new
ball game. I may
even have to buy
a new pair
of trousers."
~Lester Piggott

MOTIVATIONAL MUSING

The Office Workplace, or Breeding Ground for Fat Thighs, Soft Stomachs, and Spreading Rumps

I've received a number of pleas from Kick in the Tush members desperate to find an answer to their office food situations. From coworkers (even bosses) foisting food upon them to the ubiquitous parties—it's just too much. What has happened to the workplace? Is it just a breeding ground for fat thighs, soft stomachs, spreading rumps, and sugar highs?

Dear Our Lady of Weight Loss,

Office food is doing me in. I just don't know what to do about the birthdays, going away parties, promotion celebrations, not to mention the leftovers from the in-house meetings and luncheons, as well as the bowls and bags of candies, cookies, and chips at every turn of the cubicle. This week promises to be loaded with the inevitable fattening foods, ranging from greasy pizza to chocolate seven-layer cake and/or champagne, where I feel obligated to be polite and partake. And the culture is such that everyone comes in early, goes home late, and eats most of their meals at their desks. I haven't seen sunlight in two months. My hands are sticky with M&Ms. (I thought that they don't melt in your hands?) Please help! ~Sticky Fingers

What to Do?

Our Lady of Weight Loss to the rescue.

There are ways for us to fight the office food demons, the food and people—aka saboteurs (listed below)—and the corporate food culture.

Let's start with the Office Manifesto, a document that you can clip, paste, print, sign, and sweetly hand (minus the M&M fingerprints) to your boss.

Tasty Tidbit **Productivity faToids for Big Boss**

Those who indulge in poor eating and exercise habits account for over $33 billion in medical costs, of which $9 billion is in lost productivity due to heart disease, cancer, stroke, and diabetes.

Workdays lost for reasons related to obesity: 39.3 million

Physician office visits related to obesity: 62.7 million

Restricted activity days related to obesity: 239.0 million

Bed days related to obesity: 89.5 million.

If you do not feel comfortable printing, signing, and handing the Office Manifesto to Big Boss, you could mail it to him/her anonymously with the Office Manifesto attached. At the very least, it will raise the big boss's awareness. Next time there's an office gathering, the big boss will be noting that there's not a healthy peach in sight.

In the meantime, here are a couple of tips on how to survive the office eating culture. Once again, it takes commitment and planning—but it is worth it.

The Office Manifesto

We, the employees of _____, declare that the **state of office eating** is heretofore declared **out of control**. We hereby state the following policy.

HENCEFORTH, healthy options are to be made available at in-house meetings and parties.

HENCEFORTH, the refrigerator that the company so graciously and generously stocks with soda (both diet and regular) shall also house natural fruit juices and bottled water(s).

HENCEFORTH, the vending machine shall make available small packages of fat-free pretzels and baked potato chips.

HENCEFORTH, the "take a twenty minute break" policy will be enforced. All employees who have missed lunch and not seen the light of day are hereby required to take a twenty-minute break. It's not healthy to work without a break or to stay inside all day long.

HENCEFORTH, there will be a designated meditation/rest space(s) for employees to take refuge in during their twenty-minute breaks (in case of inclement weather).

HENCEFORTH, there will be a designated walking track (route) throughout the office. It's not healthy not to move all day long.

HENCEFORTH, no pushers are allowed. If someone says "No, thank you," the pushers shall refrain from saying "Oh, just one piece."

HENCEFORTH, the employer acknowledges that all employees are valued and said employer is thrilled to know that productivity and morale will soar if said employee is healthfully fed, gets air, and rests. ("Oh, my—such an easy solution. Thank you, Our Lady of Weight loss," says Big Boss.)

_____
Signed
_____
Date

- Just say no. There are many of us who cannot stop after one bite. If we don't say "No, thanks," we run the risk of being the size of a zeppelin.

- Have a sliver. If it's impossible to say "No, thank you" each and every time, you may want to plan to have a small piece, as in a sliver. However, if there are multiple parties per week, you may want to limit your one sliver to one party.

- Bring your own. This is what I did when I worked in a corporation that tried to ply me with food at every turn (those saboteurs!). Stock the office freezer with diet treats. From preportioned, low-fat, low-cal ice cream treats to low-cal preportioned boxed cake to 94 percent fat-free popcorn.

- Get up and move. What kind of craziness is this? Eating at your desk or not eating at all is unhealthy and contributes to fatigue and lack of concentration. Productivity drops. If you can't get out of the office, get up and walk around a couple of times. Take the long way, the stairs, or copy one piece of paper at a time.

- Take a brain break. Working without a break is unhealthy as well. Your brain goes on autopilot. Once again, productivity drops. Meditate. If you have to (I did), go to the ladies' room and close your eyes for five minutes. Do some deep breathing exercises.

- Drink more water. Drinking really helps. We often think we are hungry, when, in fact, we are actually thirsty. Try flavoring a 1.5 liter bottle of water with a little Crystal Light. And all that water provides an opportunity to go to the bathroom and meditate!

- Find a buddy. Support and company is always a good thing. Find someone to join you and you can buck the system together.

- Rebuff a food gift. When someone gives you a box of chocolate or a spaghetti pie (someone gave a Kick member one), and they know that you are trying to lose weight, refrain from hurting them. Simply smile and say, as you push the spaghetti pie back in their direction, "Oh, thanks so much, but you know, spaghetti pies aren't a part of my food plan. I appreciate the thought and would really love some fresh fruit. Why not bring it tomorrow?"

- Keep an Our Lady of Weight Loss Altar nearby. Her special powers are beyond belief. She'll change your life.

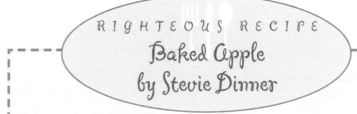

RIGHTEOUS RECIPE
Baked Apple
by Stevie Dinner

Stevie is a graduate of the Culinary Institute of America. He's a pastry chef and has maintained a forty-five-pound loss for years! Wow. If Stevie Dinner can do it, so can you!

Ingredients
¼ cup brown sugar
1½ tsps. cinnamon
rind from one lemon
4 tart apples, washed and cored
juice from one lemon

Directions

Preheat oven to 375°.

Mix brown sugar with cinnamon and lemon rind.

Place cored apples in an 8" x 8" pan.

Distribute sugar mixture evenly inside the cored apples.

Pour ½ cup boiling water into pan (not on the apples—in the pan!).

Squeeze lemon and add juice to pan.

Bake apples for about 30 minutes or until soft, not mushy, basting every 10 minutes.

Thanks, Stevie Dinner!

Nutrition Facts

Serving Size (149g)
Servings Per Container 4

Amount Per Serving

Calories 110	Calories from Fat 0

	% Daily Value*
Total Fat 0g	0%
Saturated Fat 0g	0%
Trans Fat 0g	
Cholesterol 0mg	0%
Sodium 5mg	0%
Total Carbohydrate 29g	10%
Dietary Fiber 4g	16%
Sugars 23g	
Protein 0g	

Vitamin A 2%	•	Vitamin C 15%
Calcium 2%	•	Iron 4%

*Percent Daily Values are based on a 2,000 calorie diet. Your daily values may be higher or lower depending on your calorie needs:

	Calories	2,000	2,500
Total Fat	Less Than	65g	80g
Saturated Fat	Less Than	20g	25g
Cholesterol	Less Than	300mg	300 mg
Sodium	Less Than	2,400mg	2,400mg
Total Carbohydrate		300g	375g
Dietary Fiber		25g	30g

Calories per gram:
Fat 9 • Carbohydrate 4 • Protein 4

Kick #42

Our Lady of Etiquette

"One of the greatest victories you can gain over someone is to beat him at politeness."

~Josh Billings

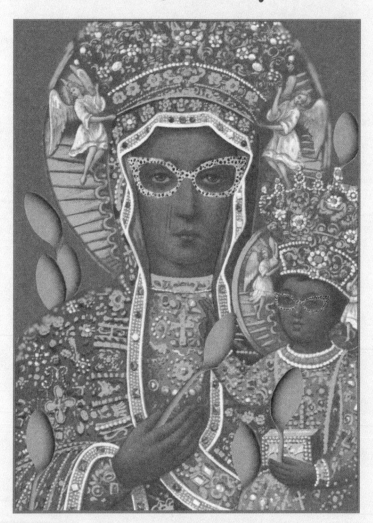

Which Spoon?

faToid

The word *present* is
preferable on formal
occasions to the word
introduce. The correct
formal introduction is:
"Our Lady of Weight
Loss, may I present
Sir Devil Cake?"

I was flicking through the television channels the other night—all one thousand of them—when I came across Julia Roberts and Richard Gere in the movie *Pretty Woman.* It was the scene in which Julia and Richard (what were their movie names?) were dining at a very fancy restaurant with the shipping magnate (played by Ralph Bellamy) and his son. Julia had no idea which fork to use, how to butter her bread, or which glass was hers, much less the proper way to eat escargots. She could get away with it—after all, she's Julia Roberts.

But it got me wondering, how might I fare in a similar situation? I mean, if I were out to dinner with Richard Gere and I sent my snail flying across the restaurant, would he still love me?

Just in case you find yourself out to dinner with a movie star, Our Lady wanted me to pass the following etiquette tips on to you.

A Baker's Dozen

Etiquette tidbits from Our Lady of Weight Loss, the patron saint of permanent fat removal

1. **Sit down.** Not so fast. After your host/hostess sits. Follow her lead.
2. **The napkin.** Now that you are seated, you should—within seconds—open the napkin and place it on your lap. Do not tuck it into your shirt, or if you've got a tie on, do not take your tie and

throw it over your shoulder. (Did I really have to tell you that?) Do not try to snap it open, either. Never leave your napkin on the table. If you need to leave the table, fold your napkin and place it on your seat.

3. **The holy bread basket.** Take a knife and cut a piece from the loaf. Take some butter and put it on your plate, not on the bread. Tear a bite-size piece of bread from the bread that you just cut and put on your plate. Butter it from your newly formed butter pile. Eat it. Repeat if you like. One piece at a time.

4. **The utensils.** Use them from the outside in. Each utensil corresponds with a course, so if you skip the first course, skip the first utensil. Never ever let a used utensil hit the table.

5. **The water glass.** It's always to your right. The dinner roll is to your left. (Hint: They're in alphabetical order: roll/water. Get it?)

6. **The soup.** Do not put the entire spoon in your mouth. Rather, fill your spoon about 75 percent with soup, bring it to your mouth, and sip it from the side.

7. **The meat (or chicken or fish).** Start from one end or the other, never in the middle, and cut one piece at a time. Have you ever seen anyone cut all their meat, potato, and vegetables, put the knife down, and chow down? Very gauche.

8. **Sit up straight.** Do not let your elbows touch the table.

9. **Pass the salt (and the pepper).** When someone asks for the salt, pass the two together. And don't salt your food until you've tasted it first. It's an insult to the cook.

10. **Chew your food.** And please, not with your mouth open. Do not talk with food in your mouth. Chew, swallow, then speak.

11. **You're a mess.** Did you spill something? Drop your napkin on the floor? Burp? Don't make a big deal over it. Stay calm. Quietly apologize. In other words, confess and move on.

12. **Finger food.** If you're not sure whether you should eat something with your fingers, opt for a utensil, but here's a short list.

   artichokes

   asparagus (only if it's without sauce)

   bacon (only if it's crisp)

   sandwiches (duh)

   cookies (duh)

   small fruits or berries with stems

   burgers, dogs, corn on the cob (obviously)

   caviar

   pickles

13. **The spectacular ending:** Place your knife and fork on the plate so that they are parallel to each other and on a diagonal—pointing toward the eleven o'clock position. Do not place them in the X position. The X indicates that you are resting between bites.

When everyone has finished their meal, you may place your napkin on the table, next to your plate, loosely—not tied in a funny knot or twisted.

Tasty Tidbit Escargots, the French word for snails, is an appetizer dish of cooked land snails. Typically, the snails are removed from their shells, gutted, and cooked (usually with garlic butter). They are then poured back into the shells, with the butter and sauce for serving. Special snail tongs (for holding the shell) and snail forks (for extracting the meat) are generally provided.

Dear Our Lady of Weight Loss,

When my son got married a few years ago, I lost thirty pounds for the occasion. Unfortunately, I gained it back. I cannot seem to get myself into the state of mind that ignites a change of lifestyle. My cousin, who is more like a sister to me, lost a lot of weight and kept it off. She's never once "tsk tsk'd" me or made me feel like a failure. I very much appreciate her not saying anything that would make me feel bad about myself. And I kind of don't want to open up that can of worms, but maybe, since she's been successful, I should ask her what her secret to success is. What do you think? ~Your avid fan . . . Nadeva, White Plains, New York

Dear Nadeva,

First things first: You're not a failure. Most people take more than one go-around to keep it off. Was this the first go-around for your cousin/sister? I'd bet not. And most people who lose weight solely for an occasion gain it back. Once the occasion has passed, where's the motivation? When people want to remove excess weight permanently they need to do it for themselves—not for anyone else, not for an occasion. You should definitely talk to your cousin/sister. I'm sure she'd be flattered.
~Our Lady of Weight Loss

Pious Project
FOOD FOR THOUGHT NAPKIN RINGS

It's always nice to end the day with a hot cup of tea. Relaxing, delicious, and if caffeine free, you've managed to get in another glass of water. Yogi Tea's Healing Formulas are among my favorites. They're really good and they have cool labels and fun tea bags with thoughtful sayings on them. They are perfect for recycling into Food for Thought Napkin Rings. A great conversation piece that provides some food for thought before we chow down.

Here's how to make a set for your next dinner party.

  paper towel cardboard tube
  small paint brush or sponge brush
  gold acrylic paint
  tea bags and tea wrappings
  craft glue
  glitter pen

INSTRUCTIONS

Cut paper towel tube into six even pieces (for six napkin rings). Paint each piece, inside and out, with gold acrylic paint. Rip off the packaging that holds the individual tea bag and glue it onto the napkin ring. (I always glue on my stuff on slightly off center.)

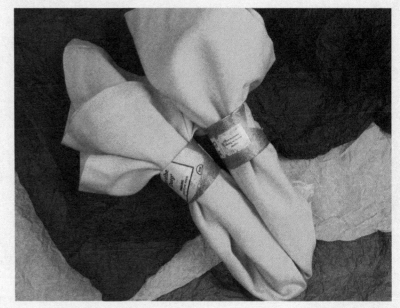

Next glue the tea bag tag with the saying onto the opposite side of the napkin ring. This one says "If we practice listening, we become intuitive." (Now that's food for thought!) Take the glitter pen and paint a little around the labels. This is a simple version. Feel free to embellish it as you like, with pearls, sequins, whatever!

Gratitude

One thing I learned for sure: We can either be collectors of injustices—feeling slighted, empty, and unhappy because of all of the injustices that have fallen upon us (both real and imagined) or we can count our blessings, feel joyful and happy, and cultivate gratitude.

Our Lady of Weight Loss hopes that you will choose the latter. She knows that there are times when it feels as if there was nothing to be grateful for. But if you take a good look, you'll find that there's always something to be appreciative of, even if it's just that you got through the day. Acknowledging the blessings in your life feels good and it opens you up to more blessings.

Our Lady encourages you to practice gratitude. Every night before you go to sleep, jot down at least five things that you are grateful for. You can use an old school notebook or even make your own! You can color code your book—

different colors for different types of blessings—you can incorporate stickers or rubber stamps into your book—anything that brings a smile to your face. Eating is often about feeding an emotion or filling a void. Perhaps the void isn't as deep as you think.

At first, you may be grateful for the obvious—food, shelter, and clothing—and then, as you strengthen your gratitude muscle, you'll find that your life is filled with more blessings than you realized. Perhaps a kind smile from a stranger will hold more meaning for you.

I am grateful that Our Lady of Weight Loss is with me. She has brought such joy and purpose to my life. She has introduced me to the most amazing people from all walks of life, from every corner of the globe.

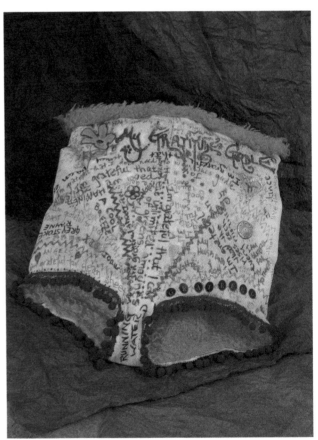

And best of all, Our Lady has made it possible that I no longer need to wear this. With love and gratitude, I dedicate this special Pious Project—My Gratitude Girdle—to Our Lady of Weight Loss.

If writing in journals is not your style, dig deep in your chest of drawers and find that old girdle, grab a bunch of fabric pens, glitter tape, orange fur—whatever!—and fill it with gratitude.

Disclaimer

I am not a doctor, nurse, nutritionist, or dietician. I'm not even a gourmet cook.

I am a regular person who—with the help of Our Lady of Weight Loss—has maintained a fifty-pound weight loss for over five years.

Our Lady of Weight Loss asked me to share my weight-loss experience with you. To the best of my knowledge, the information presented in this book is accurate. No parts of its contents should be construed as medical advice.

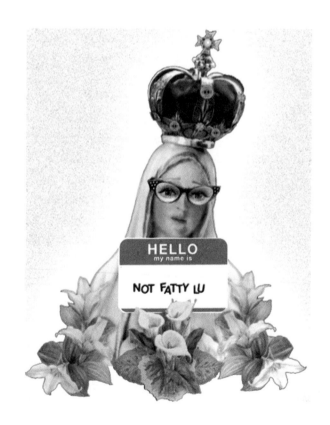

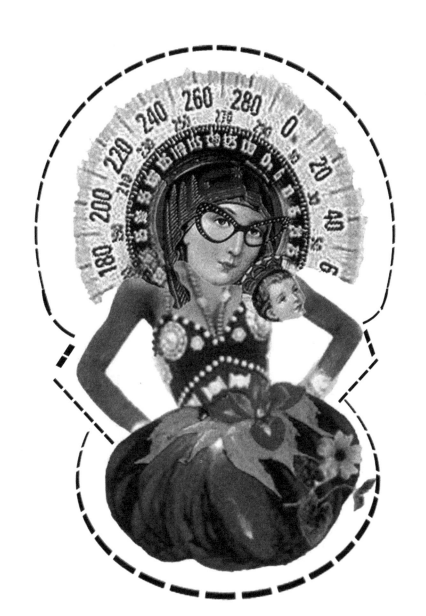

Janice Taylor is a professional weight-loss coach and America's premier weight-loss artist. A weight-loss artist is someone who makes art about food instead of eating it and, in the process, loses weight. In fact, she invented the profession.

Prior to becoming a weight-loss artist, Taylor studied textile, floral, and jewelry design and fine art. She exhibited in galleries from New York to Los Angeles to Berlin. She was also a lifelong yo-yo dieter whose favorite food group was fried.

Taylor's epiphany came one day in 2001, when she dragged herself to a weight-loss center "where people obsess about food and weight," she recalled. "I weighed in and nearly keeled over. The scales of injustice were heavy indeed. It was all so dreary and depressing. I thought, 'I'm never going to make it.'"

That is until she heard The Voice—the voice she later dubbed Our Lady of Weight Loss: *If you think you're never going to make it, you never will. You're an artist. Make weight loss an art project.* And she did, becoming America's first weight-loss artist. By connecting with her "inner thinner core" Taylor permanently removed more than fifty pounds of excess baggage.

Now Taylor writes a weekly e-newsletter, *The KICK in the TUSH Club,* at www.ourladyofweightloss.com, that shares Our Lady of Weight Loss's ideas for redirecting feeding frenzies into healthy pursuits. The *Daily News* has declared KICK a "hot trend." *Family Circle, Good Housekeeping, First for Women,* and *Good Morning America* recommended the newsletter as the place to go for weight-loss inspiration and motivation.

"Losing weight is about exploring a new way of being," Taylor said. "It's about finding creative ways to be your absolute best, and I want to help as many people realize that as possible."

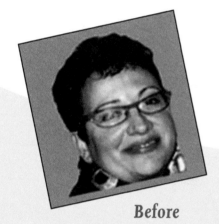

Before

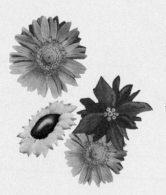

After

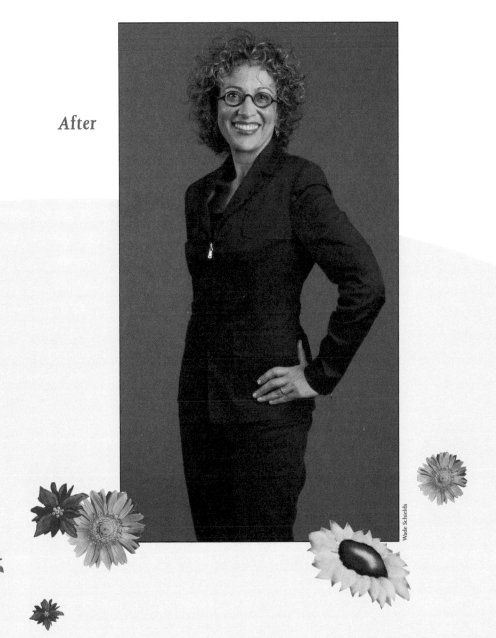

Wade Schields

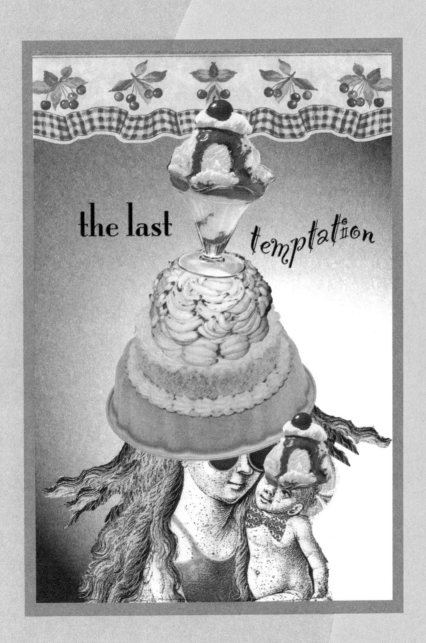